The Diagnosis and
Primary Care of Accidents and
Emergencies in Children

The Diagnosis and
Primary Care of Accidents and
Emergencies in Children

*a manual for the casualty officer
and the family doctor*

Cynthia M. Illingworth FRCP

*Consultant in Paediatric Accident and Emergency
The Children's Hospital, Sheffield*

Second Edition

Blackwell Scientific Publications

OXFORD LONDON EDINBURGH
BOSTON MELBOURNE

© 1978, 1982 by
Blackwell Scientific Publications
Editorial offices:
Osney Mead, Oxford, OX2 0EL
8 John Street, London, WC1N 2ES
9 Forrest Road
  Edinburgh, EH1 2QH
52 Beacon Street, Boston
  Massachusetts 02108, USA
99 Barry Street, Carlton
  Victoria 3053, Australia

First published 1978
Second edition 1982

Set by Santype Ltd, Salisbury
and printed by Book Plan Ltd
Worcester and London

DISTRIBUTORS

USA
  Blackwell Mosby Book
  Distributors, 11830 Westline
  Industrial Drive, St Louis
  Missouri 63141

Canada
  Blackwell Mosby Book
  Distributors, 120 Melford Drive
  Scarborough, Ontario, M1B 2X4

Australia
  Blackwell Scientific Book
  Distributors, 214 Berkeley Street
  Carlton, Victoria 3053

British Library
Cataloguing in Publication Data

Illingworth, Cynthia M.
  The diagnosis and primary care of
  accidents and emergencies in
  children.
  1. Pediatric emergencies
  I. Title
  618.92'0025   RJ370

  ISBN 0-632-00946-2

Contents

Preface to second edition, vii

Preface to first edition, ix

PART 1

General principles, 3
The challenge of Casualty, 3
There is no place for over-confidence, 3
Note-keeping, 5
Attitudes to parents, children and others, 5
History-taking, 6
Examination, 7
Special investigations, 9

Interpretation, 10
Treatment, 12
Prophylactic antibiotics, 13
Immunization against tetanus, 14
Local anaesthesia, 15
Non-accidental injury (child abuse), 16
Children brought in dead or dying, 23
If you have to go to court, 25

PART 2

Poisoning, 29
Coma, 38
Hypoglycaemia, 39
Hyperglycaemia, 39
Convulsions, 41
Lacerations, 45
Foreign bodies, 48
Burns and scalds, 55
Heat-stroke, 57
Cold injury, 59
Drowning and immersion hypothermia, 60
Cardiac and respiratory arrest, 62

Acute heart failure, 65
Severe acute asthma, 65
Anaphylaxis, 66
Road-traffic accidents, 67
Head injury, 68
Haematoma of the scalp, 73
Babies with a swelling on the scalp, 73
Injuries of the facial bones, 73
Thoracic injuries, 75
Abdominal injury, 76
The teeth, 77
The eyes, 78

Limb injuries, 83
Wringer and spin-dryer injuries to the arms, 92
Pulled elbow, 93
Trapped fingers and
 amputated fingertips,
 94

Mitten injuries, 97
Gynaecological injury, 98
Criminal injury, 98
Stings and bites, including
 rabies, 98

PART 3

Introduction, 105
Disease in immigrant
 children: illness after
 holidays abroad, 105
Any acute illness, 106
The crying baby, 107
Pyrexia of unknown origin,
 108
Acute abdominal pain, 109
Abdominal distension, 113
Vomiting, 113
Diarrhoea, 116
Blood in the stool, 119
Rectal prolapse, 119
The skin, 120
 Nappy rash, 120
 Scabies, 121
 Papular urticaria, 122
 'Hand, foot and mouth'
  disease, 124
 Chicken-pox, 124
 Molluscum contagiosum,
  125
 Bullous eruptions, 125

Exfoliative dermatitis, 125
Impetigo, 125
Boils, 126
Pediculosis capitis (nits),
 126
Purpura, 127
Sunburn, 128
Erythema nodosum, 128
Other skin conditions, 129
Other causes of Pruribus,
 130
Oedema, 130
Swelling of the face, 131
Headache and neurological
 symptoms, 132
Symptoms in the ear, nose
 and throat, 135
Some respiratory symptoms,
 138
Some genitourinary
 symptoms, 140
Limp and limb pains, 142
Swelling of a joint: arthritis,
 144

APPENDICES

Blood pressure, weight and
 height, 149

Normal values, 150
General further reading, 152

Index, 153

Preface to second edition

In revising this book I have adhered to my determination to keep it an essentially practical manual, based on many years personal experience of accident and emergency in an extremely busy department of a children's hospital. I have gone carefully through the whole text and made many alterations and additions. A few sections have been rewritten completely. With the increased risk of children abroad on holiday being bitten by rabid animals I have included a section on rabies.

I still believe that the enormous variety of medical, surgical and social problems which make up the work of a paediatric accident and emergency department make it a fascinating, challenging and instructive place to work for any doctor who wants to learn paediatrics.

Preface to first edition

This book, based on long practical experience of accident and emergency work in a busy teaching hospital, is intended primarily for 'casualty officers': but much of what is said applies equally well to the work of the family doctor. It is definitely not intended to be a comprehensive book on paediatric emergencies, many of which more concern intensive care units or the hospital ward. It is difficult or impossible adequately to draw the line between the responsibility of the accident and emergency doctor, and that of the intensive care unit: the 'flying squad' from this unit is immediately available to come to the accident and emergency department. But I have tried to delineate the responsibility of the doctor in 'Casualty'. For the family doctor, who is more responsible for primary care, much of what I have written is highly relevant. I have tried throughout to say what the doctor should not attempt to treat himself, and to name those conditions for which he must seek expert advice.

I have tried to make this book practical and explicit. I have always believed that in the case of disease, it is inadequate merely to describe the clinical picture of a disease: one should draw attention to the important variations from the usual clinical picture. For instance, it is not enough to describe the clinical picture of appendicitis or intussusception in a child; that can be read in innumerable books. It is of equal or greater importance to emphasize the variations—the occurrence, for instance, of diarrhoea in either condition, instead of the expected constipation, and in the case of intussusception the occasional absence of any pain at all.

In referring to the doctor working in an accident and emergency department, I have sometimes referred to him as the 'casualty doctor' and used the old term 'casualty department'.

The experience to be gained in a busy casualty department, in which a consultant is in full-time charge and responsible for teaching those who are more junior, is of immense value to a doctor whose aim is to specialize in general practice, community or hospital paediatrics.

I have tried to avoid describing in detail conditions in which the management is precisely the same as in adults; inevitably there must be some degree of overlap, but in children's accident and emergency work there is much less emphasis on serious trauma and much more on medical emergencies, social emergencies and the whole range of things which constitute an 'emergency' in the eyes of the parents of a young child.

I am indebted to my husband for his advice; to Mrs Valerie Sewell and Mrs Sandra Parfitt for typing the script so competently; to Mr Thorne (of 3M) for allowing me to adapt some sketches showing the method of applying Steristrip, and to the Photographic Department of the United Sheffield Hospitals for their help.

Part 1

General principles
  The challenge of Casualty
  There is no place for over-confidence
  Note-keeping
  Attitudes to parents, children and others
  History-taking
  Examination
  Special investigations
  Interpretation
  Treatment
  Prophylactic antibiotics
  Immunization against tetanus
  Local anaesthesia
Non-accidental injury (child abuse)
Children brought in dead or dying
If you have to go to court

General principles
The challenge of Casualty

A doctor working in an accident and emergency department is presented with a tremendous challenge. He is faced with a constantly varying series of problems concerning every part of the body and almost every speciality. Though much of his work is with trivial conditions which in less developed countries would never be seen by a doctor, he never knows when interspersed with trivialities there will be a major problem demanding all his skill and judgement. He feels that he is expected to know everything, and that if anything goes wrong it is he who will get the blame. At times he will be far too busy, and overwhelmed with work which is often highly exhausting—and it is when he is tired that mistakes are liable to be made; when he is hurried and pressed he forgets to record his findings in the notes, and the omission may prove to be all-important. He has constantly to use clinical judgement, but often the doctor is a junior lacking the experience necessary for good judgement. It is partly for this reason that the medical defence organizations frown on the employment of pre-registration house officers in Casualty, except when they are under the immediate supervision of a more senior doctor. However busy the casualty doctor is, he should never refuse to see a patient, for what may superficially appear to be trivial may on examination prove to be more serious.

For a doctor who is going to enter general practice, or aspires to be a paediatrician, a general physician, or a specialist in any of many other subjects, there is no better place to acquire experience than a busy accident and emergency department.

It is hoped that many will be so interested in the work that they will aim at making their future career in this area.

There is no place for over-confidence

A wise doctor never hesitates to seek advice from others, and in particular to use whatever expertise is available to him. It is

3

vital that a doctor should know when he does not know. Innumerable mistakes are made because readily available expert advice was not sought. In an accident and emergency department an experienced sister or staff nurse can provide invaluable advice, if asked; and no doctor should feel that he is 'losing face' if he asks for her opinion. In fact there is hardly a better way for the doctor to secure friendly co-operation than to make the nursing staff feel that their special experience is recognized and that they should not hesitate to express their opinion about diagnosis and management, whether that opinion is asked for or not.

In a hospital the doctor has expert advice readily available: he should use it. He should seek advice when faced with the diagnosis of a crying baby or acute abdominal pain, the management of dislocations and any but the most trivial fractures, burns or septic fingers. He should seek help when there may be difficulty in removing a foreign body from the eye, nose, ear or other orifice; and he should not attempt to remove any but the most readily accessible foreign body from the hand, foot or buttock. He should know that certain symptoms, above all others, are of particular importance in children and that failure to recognize these, with resultant failure to seek help from an expert, and particularly failure to follow up a child with one of these symptoms, is a major cause of medico-legal problems concerning children. An analysis of the mismanagement of childhood symptoms which led to claims to a medical defence organization showed that the most important conditions leading to litigation were as follows: diarrhoea, vomiting, abdominal pains, headache, convulsions and stridor. All of these will be discussed in the pages which follow.

Do not be over-confident. Do see the child again, unless that is obviously unnecessary—in an hour or two, or next day, or at a longer interval if indicated.

It would certainly not be sensible to see a child only once for stridor, vomiting, diarrhoea or any of the above symptoms, and leave to the parents the responsibility of seeing you again if the child is unwell.

If anything goes wrong, the parents in such circumstances may deny that they were told to come back if the child is unwell; in any case it is unfair to put the responsibility on the parents.

If a medico-legal problem results, the parents' statement is likely to be believed, unless a note has been made of the instruction given.

If you see a child in the hospital, it is your responsibility to use your judgement with regard to communicating with the family doctor, by letter, or if necessary by telephone. It is the duty of the hospital to provide the necessary secretarial help.

Note-keeping

Good note-keeping is essential, and the notes should be signed; the trouble is that pressure of work may make it difficult. Medical defence organizations have to pay out scores of thousands of pounds because poor note-keeping makes it impossible to provide a proper defence against such claims. When a senior person is asked for his opinion, it is desirable to ask him to write his opinion in the notes and to sign it.

It is important that the casualty notes should be kept together, and not scattered through the hospital with notes made in other departments. It is wise to arrange for a copy of the casualty notes to be incorporated with other hospital records, for otherwise the important casualty notes may be lost.

It is particularly important that all a child's attendances are kept together because the picture given when there have been several visits with bruises, a scald, an ingestion or several trivial injuries, is different from seeing the child each time as a new patient.

Attitudes to parents, children and others

It is always important but sometimes difficult to be patient and courteous to parents, particularly when one is hard-pressed, overloaded with work, irritated by them or, in a case of child abuse, angered by what they have done. When parents are in a state of panic after an accident to their child (whether it appears trivial or not to the doctor), they may be irrational, impatient, aggressive and thoroughly difficult. They may feel guilty because the accident has happened, and over-react by showing excessive anxiety. If a child is badly behaved, dirty, aggressive and displaying fear and panic unsuitable for his age, it is not easy for the doctor to remain patient and tolerant with him.

A good mother is anxious: her anxieties should always be treated seriously.

A mother who insists that there is something wrong with her child, even though the doctor can find nothing, is almost certain to be right. *It is always wrong to tell a mother that she is just over-anxious, or fussing over nothing.* It is bound to antagonize her, and in any case it is usually unjustified. A common cause of litigation is the antagonization of parents, and their feeling that they have not been kept informed, that they have been treated without due consideration for their feelings.

It must be particularly worrying for immigrant parents who cannot speak English, when they bring their child to the doctor and are unable to tell him what they fear.

History-taking

The first essential in history-taking is that each, doctor and parent or child, should understand what the other means. In paediatrics one comes to rely so much on what the parents say that one tends to forget to take the history from the child. It often happens that the child, especially if the mother is not present, reveals the true diagnosis, which the mother's history would fail to give. It is often wise to see the mother without the child, and vice versa. One lets the mother give her story, then goes back on everything that she has said to make sure that one has obtained the correct history, and for every symptom determines exactly when it was first noticed. One must always ask, 'When was the child last perfectly well?' to get a baseline for the present symptoms, whether of illness, poisoning or possible trauma. In the case of accidents one asks the exact nature of the accident, the exact time at which it happened, and exactly how it happened. This is particularly important in the case of poisoning. History-taking must be precise and as accurate as it can be. There is no place for the words 'recently' and 'frequently' without definition. If a child is said to have a raised temperature, one asks whether it was taken and by whom, and what it was. If there is said to be weight loss, one asks for the figures—and asks whether the child was clothed or not when weighed. If there is said to have been a discharge from the ears, one needs to know what the discharge was: it is usually wax. One needs to know whether there has been any relevant (especially similar) illness in the family: this is most important in the case of possible infections.

One needs to know what drugs the child has received, including those purchased without prescription from the chemist's shop. Parents commonly do not regard aspirin as a medicine or drug, and the fact that the child has been given aspirins may be important. The great frequency of side-effects of drugs must always be remembered. In his book on *Common Symptoms of Disease in Children*, Illingworth (1982) found that of the 150 common symptoms described in the book, at least 135 could be side-effects of drugs. It is also useful to know what drugs the mother and father are taking: tranquillizing and similar drugs may cloud a parent's consciousness and may be the indirect cause of a child taking some poison or becoming involved in an accident.

Examination

Every case presenting to a casualty department must be seen by a doctor. One should not rely on the judgement of a nurse. For instance, an apparently trivial cut on a finger may involve a tendon, or there may be a foreign body, such as glass, in the wound. In any case of other than obviously localized trauma, the whole child must be examined, and examined completely undressed.

The small child is likely to be afraid and anxious. He must not be allowed to see other injured children or anything unpleasant to alarm him. By suitable conversation with him much of his fear can be allayed. Talk to him and keep talking to him. Encourage the mother to keep talking to him.

The first part of the examination is made on his mother's knee if he is a small child, or at least with his mother holding him. One notes the state of nutrition, height, hydration, and any rashes, blemishes, bruises or scars, and *writes them in the notes.*

A toddler commonly objects strongly to lying down, in which case the abdomen can be examined when he is kneeling or standing. A toddler will often stop crying when his vest is put on, and the rest of the examination can then be completed. When examining the abdomen the well-trained doctor does not keep his eyes on the umbilicus but on the child's face, watching to determine whether there is tenderness. One does not ask him if it hurts, suggesting that it does; one watches him. When examining for enlargement of the spleen, the head should rest on a low pillow; if the head is raised farther, the tip of an enlarged spleen will be missed.

When there are abdominal symptoms, one must examine the hernial orifices and the genitalia. It is easy to miss a torsion of the testis if the pants are left on.

Areas of discomfort are left to the last: if he limps on the right leg, one examines the other leg first. If he is just 'not very well', the examination is not complete unless his skin is thoroughly inspected for a rash or petechiae, and the buccal mucosa for Koplik's spots. The lower eyelid is examined for petechial haemorrhages. The palms of the hand and the sole of the foot are examined for the vesicular rash of 'hand, foot and mouth' disease. The mouth is also examined for herpes stomatitis.

If after an accident there is an obvious swelling or deformity of a limb, one avoids unnecessary examination if an X-ray is obviously necessary, but remember the importance of checking the radial pulse and finger movements in elbow injuries. In order to assess the range of movement, one watches him playing with a toy, or gets him to follow a torch. Slight local warmth often helps to locate the site of a fracture in a toddler, e.g. a greenstick fracture of the tibia.

The examination of the mouth for tonsillitis or thrush is left until last. The older child may prefer to depress his tongue with his own finger. Neck stiffness is tested for when he is sitting up if possible, watching his face for expression of pain when one is flexing the neck.

If a rectal examination is necessary in a small child, one uses the little finger, placing it *gently* against the anus and *gently* increasing the pressure until it can be inserted without difficulty, *talking to the child all the time as it is done.* The thermometer is placed in his groin or axilla, and is left for the *full three minutes*, even if it is said to be a half-minute thermometer. Rectal temperatures are disliked by the child, carry a small risk, and are better avoided.

Special investigations

The doctor's surgery or the accident and emergency department is no place for complex investigations. The doctor has to decide at what stage to refer a child to an out-patient clinic or for admission.

With regard to X-ray examinations, the radiologist must be given the necessary information, e.g. points of maximum tenderness or swelling. There must be a system whereby the X-ray report is seen by the doctor. In medico-legal cases the casualty doctor's interpretation of an X-ray carries little weight in comparison with the radiologist's report. The defence organizations have to pay numerous claims because a radiologist's (or laboratory) report was not seen by the doctor who asked for the investigations. Digits should be described by name and not by number and 'right' and 'left' written out in full. If glass has been involved in the injury X-rays *must* be done. X-rays should only be asked for at night if it is impossible without an X-ray to decide about appropriate treatment. If it can wait until morning without harm to the patient, it is wise for medico-legal reasons to make the appropriate entry in the notes.

With regard to other laboratory investigations, those most likely to be requested, and most likely to be useful, are urine examinations for albumin, sugar, microscopy and culture. It is useless asking the parent to 'bring in a specimen of urine':

urine must be examined within a few minutes of being passed, and preferably a mid-stream specimen; if this is impossible, a dip-slide or uripot is a satisfactory alternative. *Remember that a urinary tract infection should be proved before treatment is given,* and the child should be referred to the paediatrician for investigation.

If salicylate poisoning is suspected, the phenistix test will help.

The ESR is done as a non-specific test which helps one (in part only) to eliminate an infective process or certain organic diseases. Other investigations are mainly: the haemoglobin, red cell and white cell count, and where relevant, the platelet count; simple investigations of the blood-clotting mechanism; examinations for sickling where relevant; and blood sugar, blood urea and serum electrolytes.

When a child urgently requires fluid, blood is taken for electrolytes and culture and a drip started, based on a judicious guess. When an ill child is to be admitted, it may save time if blood for the most urgent investigations, such as blood sugar, is taken in Casualty.

When a child comes to Casualty and is known to have a bleeding disorder, such as haemophilia, Christmas disease or Von Willebrand's disease, he should not be sent home without consulting the haematologist. The child should have with him a green card, stating the diagnosis.

Interpretation

Any doctor is more likely to make the correct diagnosis if he thinks of the common conditions before the rare ones, but he has to be on his guard against being misled by the obvious. For instance, when a child has a convulsion following a head injury, one has to be sure that it was not a convulsion which caused the fall and the head injury.

It is common in a casualty department to see a child who is said to be poorly following a head injury, only to find that he is poorly, not because of the head injury, but because he has otitis media or a urinary tract infection. A child may be presented as a possible case of poisoning, whereas careful history-taking and examination reveal a different cause for his symptoms, e.g. an intussusception. The presenting symptoms as given by the parents may be far removed from the real reasons for the parents' visit. They may complain that he has abdominal pain (but more frequently a wide variety of symptoms, none of them suggesting organic disease) when in fact they are afraid that the child may have the same condition as their neighbour's child, namely leukaemia—but they are afraid to voice their real fears.

A normal child was brought with a query as to whether he was 'brain-damaged' because the parents had heard on television that if a baby was cleansed with hexachlorophane it made him mentally defective; only direct questioning as to what they were really afraid of revealed the true cause of their anxiety.

An excessive display of parental anxiety may be an indication of child abuse. One has to avoid the mistake of making a simple diagnosis in the child, when the real diagnosis is serious domestic friction, or illness in the parent. When an older child repeatedly comes to the doctor without his parents, he may be playing truant from school—or displaying the Munchausen syndrome. 'Munchausen by proxy' has been described in which the parent claims that the child has symptoms which he has not, and causes those symptoms to get him into hospital, e.g. by giving him a drug to make him unconscious and concealing this action.

One must know not only the common and vitally important variations from the clinical picture of disease, but also the normal variations, and possible laboratory errors, in special investigations. For instance, it is easy to be misled by normal variations in epiphyseal growth in X-rays, so that fractures are wrongly diagnosed.

It is easy to misdiagnose as disease, symptoms due to the side-effects of drugs or to poisoning. Meningitis may be diagnosed when the symptoms and signs are those of phenothiazine toxicity. Solvent-sniffing produces a wide variety of signs and symptoms.

Referred pain is a well-known snare. In children the following are the main sources of confusion:

1   Pain in the knee, referred from hip disease, and vice versa.
2   Pain in the abdomen, referred from the chest.
3   Pain in the left shoulder, referred from a ruptured spleen.
4   Pain in the wrist or shoulder, referred from a pulled elbow.
The pain from a fracture (e.g. the tibia) may conceal an injury elsewhere (e.g. the hip).

The greatest snare, as in many other branches of medicine, is the combination of functional and organic. The presence of obvious psychological symptoms does not exclude coexisting organic disease. A mother may bring a child on frequent occasions with trivial complaints for which no cause is found but *the danger is that one day there may be a cause,* and a cause which needs urgent treatment. Recurrent abdominal pain may one day present as a volvulus or intussusception.

The important thing for the doctor is to know when he does NOT know, to seek advice where relevant and to be sure that he follows the child's progress.

Treatment

Drugs should not be prescribed except for precise indications, and not without a diagnosis being made. It is dangerous and unjustified. *For instance, the common practice of prescribing metoclopramide or prochlorperazine for a vomiting child, without making a proper diagnosis, is malpractice.*

It is equally wrong to prescribe a sedative for a crying child or for abdominal pain without making a diagnosis: it may conceal a serious abdominal emergency.

The casualty department is no place for the use of exotic antibiotics: they should not be necessary and their use should be reserved for a possible future occasion when a child really needs them and has not become allergic to them.

Polypharmacy is unnecessary, expensive and can produce dangerous side-effects. Many things clear up without drugs. Most upper respiratory tract infections are viral in origin and need no treatment.

The new edition of the *British National Formulary* is a valuable source of help. If a drug is prescribed, it should be prescribed for a specific period and then discontinued. You must make sure that the mother understands the instructions, and the length of time for which the drug has to be given. One has seen patients told to take two aspirins at night after an injury, and who were found to be still taking the drugs four months later. You must make sure that the child is not already taking medicine: this is important, for if you, too, prescribe some, he may receive an overdose, or take a medicine which affects the action of the other one.

A good doctor treats the whole child, and not merely the presenting symptoms. For instance, a child is brought in for a grazed knee, and he is noticed to be deaf or to require orthodontic treatment: the appropriate treatment should be arranged. Whatever is done, the family doctor should be informed.

No drugs should be prescribed unless the possible side-effects are known.

Before penicillin is prescribed you must ask if the child has had it before and if there were any problems associated with its use. *If he is penicillin sensitive, record this on his notes.*

Many children are sensitive to adhesive plaster and you should ask about this before it is applied to the skin.

Prophylactic antibiotics

Extensive studies have shown that the use of antibiotics for prophylaxis after injury are of little if any value. Cultures of wounds reaching the casualty department have shown surprisingly little infection (Illingworth R. S. Antibiotic prophylaxis in a children's hospital casualty department. *Practitioner* 1973; **210**: 693). Swabs taken from 107 lacerations grew significant organisms in only eight cases. If there are antibiotic-sensitive organisms, they may be destroyed, but insensitive ones are allowed to grow. It is better to deal with wounds by standard surgical techniques—by thoroughly cleaning and the removal of dead tissue and foreign matter. Perhaps the one exception is the penetrating wound which has occurred in a situation which would carry the risk of Clostridium welchii infection and which it is impossible to open up to achieve proper surgical debridement and removal of necrotic tissue. In these wounds it is wise to give penicillin to destroy organisms which may have been introduced. Tetanus prophylaxis is managed as outlined in the next section. It is important to clean parts surrounding a laceration: it would not be enough to clean the site of a laceration, for example on a hand, and leave the rest of the hand dirty. A bowl of soapy water should often precede 'surgical' cleansing.

If a wound already shows infection a swab should be taken to determine the organism and its sensitivity, and the part put at rest by a sling or other method according to its site. If it appears that the infection is not responding spontaneously, the appropriate antibiotic is given for a full course. For the haemolytic streptococcus, penicillin (not ampicillin) is given *for a full ten days*. Over 90% of staphylococcus aureus infections seen in Casualty are penicillin resistant. Cloxacillin or flucloxacillin are usually the drugs to which the organism will be sensitive. Before prescribing any penicillin preparation, one must ask whether there has been evidence of allergy to penicillin.

Immunization against tetanus

This section concerns the prevention of tetanus. When a child is seen on account of a wound, particularly a penetrating one, such as a dog bite or eye injury, one must determine his immunization status and *record it on his notes*. Remember that tetanus can also occur with burns, after dental extraction, with eye infections, discharging ears and chronic skin ulcers. If he has not been immunized against tetanus, or one cannot be sure whether he has, and protection against tetanus is advisable, he is given 250 units of human tetanus immunoglobulin (Humotet), and the first dose of diphtheria and tetanus immunization into the opposite leg. If the child is around ten years old or older, and has had no previous immunization, it is unwise to give the usual preparation used for the pre-school child, because there is a risk of an unpleasant reaction to the diphtheria components: he is given TAF and tetanus toxoid simultaneously. Send a letter to the immunization department of the local authority to arrange the rest of the course.

If he has been previously immunized, but has not had a booster or other tetanus toxoid in the last three years (some say five years), he is given a booster of tetanus toxoid. If he has had a dose of toxoid in the previous three years, he should not be given a further booster. First, it is unnecessary and second, too frequent doses of toxoid carry a risk of sensitivity reactions—angioneurotic oedema, urticaria, asthma or serum sickness. If the child is nearing the age of school entry and has not had a booster of tetanus toxoid, he is given the normal diphtheria and tetanus immunization, so that he avoids an unnecessary injection before he starts school. If possible give the polio booster too, but if no polio vaccine is available remember to tell the parents that he will still need a poliomyelitis booster on school entry. *If the parents refuse immunization, write this on the child's notes and get the parent to sign it.*

When there is a serious wound or a bad compound fracture it is wise to give anti-tetanus immunoglobulin in addition to the booster tetanus toxoid in a previously immunized child.

Local anaesthesia

Local anaesthetics are of limited use in small children and you must be prepared to ask for general anaesthetics more often than would be the case in adults. Entonox can help when the child is old enough to co-operate.

The most important thing is to *infiltrate slowly*—using the finest short needles possible, e.g. 25 G $\times$ $\frac{5}{8}$ (16 mm $\frac{5}{10}$), for the initial injection and then changing to a longer one. Vasoconstrictors should not be used in anaesthesia of digits. A dental syringe and a supply of 'dental needles' are extremely useful for giving local anaesthetic because the needles are so fine and the syringe makes the control of the injection much more precise. The only dental ampoules available without vasoconstrictors are of 2% Xylocaine so that you must remember that the quantities given must be adjusted carefully.

For local anaesthesia in and around the mouth, before

giving the initial injection, a small amount of 5% Xylocaine ointment applied on a piece of cotton wool and held in contact with the proposed injection site for five to ten minutes will make the subsequent infiltration with local anaesthetic more comfortable. Use a small short needle.

Elsewhere a small quantity of Xylocaine spray can, if necessary, be used before infiltration to reduce discomfort.

Ethyl chloride spray is useless as an anaesthetic for opening abscesses, paronychias, etc., and should under no circumstances be used for this purpose.

Non-accidental injury (child abuse)

If you are seeing many children you will find that you have to devote a considerable amount of time to social problems, of which non-accidental injury (child abuse) is a major one. Because of this, and because it is of vital importance to recognize these conditions, they will be discussed in detail.

The manifestations are so varied that you *must continually bear the possibility in mind when seeing young children.*

It may present as:

Fractures (especially in a young child).

Subdural effusion.

Bruises.

Haemorrhages in the eye, scrotum or scalp (from hair pulling).

Torn frenum of the upper lip.

Visceral injuries.

Burns.

Poisoning.

Failure to thrive.

Marks from human bites.

Apathy from severe emotional deprivation or emotional trauma.

'Always vomiting'.

'Always crying'.

Deprivation—lack of physical care or hygiene.

Many of the injuries, subdural effusion and fractures in particular, are thought to be due to shaking the child or the limb, rather than to direct physical violence.

Background

There is commonly a history of emotional deprivation and punitive disciplinary methods in the childhood of one or, worse still, both parents. The parents commonly left school early, often after truancy, the father experiencing unemployment and a poor work record, with poor housing, low income, a criminal record or alcoholism. The parents are often young: the pregnancy is often unwanted and the child illegitimate. Only a small proportion of the parents are true psychopaths. More often than in controls there is a history that the child was 'small for dates', treated in an intensive care unit at birth, with prolonged separation from the mother in hospital or subsequent separation from the parents because of illness or for social reasons. *The child is most at risk in his first three years.* He is at special risk if he is retarded, handicapped, small, ugly, the wrong sex, or if he resembles a disliked relative.

Though this is the common background to child abuse, it is a mistake to assume that such a background is invariable. *Child abuse is by no means confined to the lower social classes* but reasonable living conditions, the money to have a holiday or to pay someone to look after the child occasionally, may reduce some of the stress or make it easier to conceal the results. An important feature in any social class is a history of emotional deprivation and punitive discipline in the parents' childhood.

In any social class, precipitating factors which lead to child abuse are psychological stress, illness, fatigue or domestic friction, but particularly prolonged uncontrollable crying by the baby, or the toddler's refusal to eat or use the potty—features of the normal negativism of the one to three year old. The child cries partly because he wants to be picked up and loved: but it is made worse by smacking or otherwise punishing him, so that a vicious circle is established. The mother then feels at the end of her tether: she feels that she could scream, run away, wring the baby's neck, shake him—and perhaps she does—and then there is trouble. The dividing line between wanting to shake the baby and doing it is a slender one, and the mother is often afraid that she will lose her temper one day and do it. Her frustration is increased by the impossibility of reasoning with a young child or a crying baby and she is genuinely afraid that she will harm him. She hopes that some-one will recognize her plight, but she is afraid to confess her fear: and so she complains to the doctor that the child is 'always crying', or is 'vomiting continuously', or 'has diar-rhoea', or is retarded. The doctor has to assess the condition, take a full history and examine the child, and interpret his findings with care, before he reaches the conclusion that this is a 'pre-battering' condition, and that the mother is in urgent need of help.

Features which should arouse suspicion of non-accidental injury

The precise cause of injuries in young children may often be difficult to determine as may also the precise cause of their having been brought to a doctor. Think carefully when:

1   there has been delay between the accident happening and the parents attending for advice;
2   the story of what is said to have happened is implausible or does not fit the clinical findings;
3   there is evidence of earlier injury;
4   the mother complains that the baby is 'always crying'—and no organic cause is found;
5   the child is brought frequently for little apparent reason, e.g. is said to be 'always vomiting' when no cause is found and the child is thriving, is said to have 'constant diarrhoea' when nothing is found, etc.;
6   the child has been seen with a combination of things, e.g. minor trauma, burns, ingestions or simply frequent attend-ances;
7   there is a complaint that the child 'bruises easily'—but remember that this may be true;
8   there is vaginal bleeding and vaginal discharge in a pre-puberbal girl: this should raise the possibility of sexual ex-ploitation in addition to the obvious cause of a foreign body, so think of the possibility;
9   it is known that this is a family in which there is a situation of risk.

Examination

1 *The parents*—they may appear to be well-dressed and normal but you may notice something unusual in the attitude of the mother or father—a rejecting disinterest or perhaps excessive agitation out of proportion to the severity of the mishap. The desk clerk or nurses may notice something odd about their behaviour. The mother may perhaps have a bruise or a black eye.

2 *The child*—features on examination of the child which should arouse suspicion include:

a *Bruising.* Facial bruising, especially around the mouth. Small bruises or petechiae at the base of the neck which could be caused by holding the child when shaking him.
Bruises on the back or on *both* sides of the body in a very young child. (Do not fail to recognize mongolian pigmentation.)
Bruises of differing ages.
Bruising with a particular pattern, e.g. finger marks or linear bruises from being hit by a strap.
Marks from human bites.

b *Tearing of the frenum* of the upper lip, even though there is no external sign of injury.

c Evidence of earlier injuries.

d *Burns* or scars of previous burns.
Cigarette burns—round scars about 1 cm in diameter.
Burns which do not fit the history of the accident, e.g. on both sides of the body when the child is said to have fallen against a radiator.

e Unexplained scratches.

f Failure to thrive.

g Severe, untreated napkin rash.

h *Fractures,* especially in the first two years; about a quarter of these are thought to be due to child abuse.
A single long-bone fracture, such as a fractured femur in a three-month-old baby, is almost certainly due to non-accidental injury. There may be X-ray evidence of subperiosteal haemorrhage or periosteal elevation, metaphyseal fragmentation (commonly due to shaking the child), with new

bone formation along the shaft of long bones, or epiphyseal displacement. A spiral fracture of the humerus or femur may be caused by holding the baby by the wrist or ankle and jerking him upwards and rotating him. A transverse fracture is more likely to be due to direct violence. A spiral or transverse fracture of a long bone may be due to falling out of a cot or dropping the child out of or into a cot. There may be fractures of ribs; the commonest site is on the posterior aspect near the spine and it is often bilateral due to compression of the chest. Antero-posterior compression may fracture the ribs in the axillary line. There may also be fractures at the costochondral junctions. The presence of new bone formation means that the injury is at least seven to ten days old.

If child abuse is strongly suspected in a young child it will usually be necessary to do a skeletal survey. This decision should be made by a senior doctor because of the amount of irradiation involved.

X-rays taken seven to ten days later may show evidence of new bone formation in areas which looked normal on the original films.

The whole child should be examined thoroughly. The optic fundi should be examined for the presence of haemorrhages, even though there is no external evidence of injury to the skull.

It is important that when a child in whom non-accidental injury is thought to be a possibility is examined, that attention is paid to any signs of trauma around the anus and around the external genitals, in addition to the rest of the body. The hymen should be inspected for any redness, abrasion or purpura. In most cases of course there are no confirmatory physical findings. There may be physical signs inexplicable except as a result of child abuse. An experienced doctor or nurse sometimes just 'feels that there is something wrong' with little concrete evidence to support that feeling.

Record your findings carefully, including negative findings, e.g. after examining the perineum.

Mark on a sketch diagram the position and type of bruises and other injuries. Such a diagram, made by the examining doctor at the time, is usually easier to use as evidence in court than photographs taken by someone else, but these should also be done if possible. It is essential to record anything unusual about the history, the parental attitude, or the physical findings; this, together with an accurate record of the injuries, may help the court to decide a child's future. Confidential social information, however, should not be included in the casualty notes, but kept on a special card which can be locked away.

It would be a mistake to assume that there will always be extensive injuries in a case of child abuse. The injuries may be only trivial or there may be no injury. *The severity of the crisis or the danger to the child does not necessarily correlate with the extent or severity of the injuries. A baby brought on account of excessive crying, or with only a small facial bruise, may be in greater danger than one with several fractures.*

Differential diagnosis

The manifestations of child abuse are so protean that it would not be profitable to discuss every possible differential diagnosis. However, one must remember the obvious facts: bruising may be due to blood diseases; mongolian pigmentation on the lower sacral area and commonly on the dorsum of the ankles resembles bruises; there may be periosteal elevation in scurvy, syphilis and Caffey's syndrome of infantile cortical hyperostosis; and fractures may be related to bone disease.

Management

Consult the 'at risk' register in your area. *This may support your suspicions, but the fact that the child is not on the register does not rule out the possibility of child abuse and if you are unhappy about the situation you must deal with it appropriately. Your first responsibility is to make sure that the child is safe.* Nearly always this will mean admitting him to hospital. *Do not on any account accuse the parents of having caused the injury.* There is usually no difficulty in getting the parents' permission for the child to be admitted by saying that he has to have tests to 'see why he is bruising easily', why he is 'always falling' or why he is 'not thriving'. If you think that there is a 'pre-battering' situation, in which the child is at considerable risk, because the mother is at the end of her tether, the baby must be admitted.

Forensic examination. If there are cases in which sexual abuse or rape has been alleged it is important that a forensic pathologist helps with collecting the evidence, because this has to stand up in court. He will collect hair specimens, finger nail scrapings and sperm tests.

If the NSPCC or other social agency bring a child they are worried about, he must be admitted if proper arrangements have not already been made for his safety. *The parents must have been told by the social worker that the child is being brought to hospital and whether he is admitted.*

You must make sure that the admitting doctor is aware of the full reasons for the admission and for your concern about the child's safety, and you must make sure that the medical social worker is informed.

Unless the child is under a Place of Safety Order you have no right to prevent the parents from taking him home at any time. If the child is in danger, it is urgent to obtain an order. It can be done day or night. It can be arranged by a social worker, the NSPCC or the police. The order has to be signed by a magistrate and gives custody of the child in a 'place of safety' for 28 days. During that time a decision has to be made about all the home conditions and whether or not the case will be taken to the Juvenile Court to try to get a 'Care Order' for the child. This must be done before the end of the 28 days unless an extension is applied for. Once the Place of Safety Order has expired, if a Care Order has not been obtained or no extension of the Place of Safety Order, the parents have the right to remove the child.

The legal aspects of childhood injury and neglect were well summarized in an article by Black and Hughes (*Br. med. J.* 1979, **ii**:910).

Hospital records and photographs are the property of the hospital and must not be released by a junior doctor to anyone outside the hospital.

There are voluntary organizations which offer help to parents who are feeling that they may injure their children.

Summary

1   Think carefully about any attendance by a young child and in particular about facial bruising, unusual bruises elsewhere, fractures in young children, babies who are 'always crying', and young children who have attended an unusual number of times with burns, minor injuries, ingestions or any other reason.
2   Make careful records with sketches and photographs.
3   Treat the parents with care and courtesy even if you think they may have injured their child.
4   Admit the child if you are concerned about his safety or if you think there is a 'pre-battering' situation.
5   Remember that without a Place of Safety Order you have no power to prevent the parents taking the child home at any time.

Children brought in dead or dying

The practice of examining a child in the ambulance in order to determine whether or not he is dead is an unsatisfactory procedure and it may lead to a false assumption of death, e.g. in a child suffering from profound hypothermia. If a child is brought to the hospital by the ambulance service it does imply that there is some doubt about whether or not he is alive and in that case the child should be brought in so that he can be examined properly and in satisfactory conditions.

When a child is brought in dead or dies a few minutes after arriving at the hospital after unsuccessful attempts at resuscitation, there is a particularly distressing situation not only for the parents but for the professional staff who are concerned.

The problem concerns mainly infants of a few months of age who have been found dead in the cot or pram ('cot deaths' or 'sudden infant death syndrome').

A few children are brought in dead or dying after an accident—some in the terminal stage of an already diagnosed disease, some as a result of an acute condition such as meningo-coccal septicaemia or poisoning, and some as a result of some condition which has not previously been recognized. *Remember the possibility, especially in an infant, of non-accidental injury.*

The history should be taken from the parent or parents while resuscitation attempts are made if these are indicated. This should include neonatal illnesses, recent or otherwise, and drugs taken by the child. The parents should not be left alone to feel isolated and forgotten in their distress.

In the case of a 'cot death', the rectal temperature should be taken and the exact time recorded. Any unusual feature about the baby or the circumstances in which he was found should be included in the notes.

When the child *is* dead the parents must be told gently and kindly, and allowed to ask any questions they wish. They should be asked if they wish to see or to hold the baby. They should be told that if they would like to do this later or come back again to have further questions answered they can do so. They must be told that in any case of unexpected death the coroner has to be told and there has to be a post-mortem examination. Some of their questions can only be answered after this.

The parents must be warned that the police may visit the home but that this must not be taken as an indication that they are responsible for the death.

After speaking to the coroner's officer you should inform the family doctor and contact the hospital medical social worker so that she can help the parents in their bereavement and in their feelings of guilt and distress. In some areas there are special social workers who visit and give help to parents who have had an unexpected infant death. There are also vol-untary groups, some consisting of parents who have lost a child in similar circumstances and who will give long-term support.

The parents can be given information about the Foundation for the Study of Infant Deaths (4, 5 Grosvenor Place, London SW1X 7HD).

It is important that the health visitor and the local authority medical services know about the child's death so that further distress is not caused by sending clinic and immunization appointments for a baby who has died.

If you have to go to court

If you deal with any case in which some police or court action is possible it is particularly important that your notes made at the time are meticulous and are accompanied by diagrams and measurements of bruises, abrasions, etc., and, if possible, photographs of them.

Take a photocopy of any such notes and keep them safely, because months may go by before the case comes to court.

Before going to court

Know the facts of the case and your own findings.

Think about the questions you may be asked and how you will answer them.

Do not give opinions about things which you are not qualified to do, e.g. psychiatric opinions, because counsel may ask, 'Are you a psychiatrist?' What you can do is to describe the patient's or parents' behaviour or things said to you or in your presence—the *exact* words if possible.

Be neatly dressed and arrive on time.

Do not be afraid to say that you do not know, but be prepared to maintain what you have seen for yourself.

Part 2

Poisoning
Coma
Hypoglycaemia
Hyperglycaemia
Convulsions
Lacerations
Foreign bodies
Burns and scalds
Heat-stroke
Cold injury
Drowning and immersion hypothermia
Cardiac and respiratory arrest
Acute heart failure
Severe acute asthma
Anaphylaxis
Road-traffic accidents
Head injury
Haematoma of the scalp
Babies with a swelling on the scalp
Injuries of the facial bones
Thoracic injuries
Abdominal injury
The teeth
The eyes
Limb injuries
Wringer and spin-dryer injuries to the arms
Pulled elbow
Trapped fingers and amputated fingertips
Mitten injuries
Gynaecological injury
Criminal injury
Stings and bites, including rabies

Poisoning

Hundreds of potential poisons are available to children. In this section I shall discuss general principles and a few of the more common ingestants.

General principles

Approximately 650 children each year come to the accident and emergency department at the Children's Hospital, Sheffield, on account of poisoning.

In a study which I carried out in Sheffield in 1974 I found that the commonest poisons taken were salicylates, tranquillizers and antidepressants, especially diazepam. More careful packaging has reduced the numbers of aspirin ingestion in young children but enteric-coated and sustained-release preparations are an increasing hazard.

There is such a vast number of potential poisons that it is impossible to know the possible results of many of them. One can often determine the constituents of proprietary preparations by telephoning the makers. An alternative is to telephone the poisons centre, e.g.

Edinburgh 031-229-2477
London 01-407-7600
Leeds 0532-32799

Useful reference books are:

MARTINDALE *Extra Pharmacopoea.* 27th edn. London: Pharmaceutical Press, 1977.

NORTH P. *Poisonous Plants and Fungi.* London: Blandford Press, 1967.

VALE J.A. & MEREDITH T.J. *Poisoning: diagnosis and treatment.* London: Update Publications, 1980.

A busy casualty department should keep its own card index of common poisons, their results and treatment, and constant additions will be made to it. University botany departments and parks departments can be most helpful in identifying plants and berries which have been ingested.

You must always try to obtain the original container of fluid or

29

tablets taken. If a parent telephones for advice about a poisoning tell her to bring the container, remaining tablets, etc., with her when she brings the child.

Try to find out how many tablets or how much of the liquid has been taken, *but always assume that the child may have taken more than one is told :* on the other hand, he may have taken virtually none of it.

The symptoms and signs produced by ingested poisons (or by solvent sniffing) are so protean and sometimes so bizarre, that poisoning should always be kept in mind when an ill child is seen and one cannot positively identify the cause. On no account must you be misled by the parents' denial that the child has taken a poison: the parents may be confused, they may feel guilty because they inadvertently or deliberately left medicine accessible to the child, or they may genuinely not know, and mislead the doctor. *An overdose or other poisoning may be a manifestation of child abuse.*

Do not fall into the trap of being misled by the latent period between the ingestion of certain poisons and the development of symptoms. The most important dangerous drugs after whose ingestion the child may be symptom-free for several hours are salicylates, iron, diphenoxylate and fungi. Enteric-coated and sustained-release tablets are particularly dangerous in this respect.

Another trap consists of assuming that when a child is brought on account of poisoning, his symptoms are necessarily due to the ingestion of poison. I have seen a child brought by the parents with a confident diagnosis of poisoning because when the child looked unwell they asked him if he 'had eaten something'; examination revealed that the child's symptoms were due to intussusception.

The history

It is important to do one's best to determine what drug or other poison the child took, exactly *when* he took it, how much of it he is thought to have taken, and how he obtained it. Ask whether the mother or father is receiving drugs and therefore perhaps had a reduced level of consciousness, or carelessly left the drugs in an accessible place. Ask whether other children in the family may also have taken some of the poison; if there is any doubt the other children should be seen as well.

The examination

The whole child must be examined. If there is a possibility that the child has ingested a corrosive substance, his mouth and throat should be examined for burns.

Clothes contaminated by corrosive substances, e.g. turpentine or paint remover, must be removed and not put back on to the child. The skin must be washed immediately and thoroughly before completing the examination.

Official investigations

If an ingested poison or drug cannot be identified, and some of the remaining poison is available, it may be analysed: material aspirated from the stomach should be retained and a specimen of urine and sometimes blood should be obtained for examination. If the child has possibly ingested salicylate, iron or paracetamol the blood level can be estimated.

Interpretation

Remember the possibility of child abuse.

The symptoms and signs of poisoning are so diverse that it is not possible to attempt to list all the possible symptoms and the drugs which might have caused them. The following, however, are some of the more important symptoms in relation to commonly ingested poisons:

Excitement, hallucinations—belladonna, diphenoxylate, antihistamines, tranquillizers, alcohol, phenobarbitone, hallucinogenic toadstools (Psylocybin) and solvent sniffing.

Confusion—alcohol, antidepressants and tranquillizers, amphetamine, antihistamines, antiepileptic drugs, fenfluramine and the belladonna group.

Coma—alcohol, carbon monoxide, antiepilepsy drugs, antihistamines, tranquillizers and sedatives, haloperidol, amphetamine, salicylates, organic phosphates and thallium.

Convulsions—alcohol, amphetamines, antidepressants, tranquillizers, salicylates, antihistamines, insecticides and plants.

Torsion spasm, involuntary movements, trismus—the Phenothiazine group, metoclopramide, phenytoin, amphetamines, haloperidol, antidepressants and antihistamines.

Small pupils—opiates, diphenoxylate and organo-phosphorus insecticides.

Dilated pupils—belladonna, atropine, antihistamines, amphetamines and monoamine oxidase inhibitors (often with a delay of 12 hours or more).

Dry mouth—belladonna, atropine, antihistamines and nitrozepam.

Salivation, lachrymation—phenothiazines, organo-phosphorus insecticides, anticholinesterase eye drops (phospholine iodide), haloperidol, fungi, arsenic, mercury and thallium.

Ataxia—alcohol, antiepilepsy drugs, antihistamines, tranquillizers, solvent sniffing, diphenoxylate, piperazine and nitrazepam.

Bradycardia—digoxin, Lily of the Valley and narcotics.

Tachycardia—alcohol, atropine, ephedrine and amphetamines.

Cardiac arrhythmia—tricyclic antidepressants, chloral hydrate, potassium, digoxin, atropine and solvent sniffing.

Treatment

Except when a child is unconscious, or has ingested paraffin, petroleum distillates, kerosene, turpentine or a corrosive, it is customary to give 15 ml of syrup of ipecacuanha followed by 200 ml of water, repeated in 15 to 20 minutes if necessary. The time at which the ipecacuanha is given *must be recorded on the notes*, and whether or not the child has vomited afterwards recorded. Those with much practical experience of dealing with young children know that a negativistic toddler may strongly disapprove of syrup of ipecacuanha and it may be almost impossible to persuade him to take it; and if it is urgent

that his stomach contents should be removed, vomiting as a
result of syrup of ipecacuanha is commonly delayed for 15 to
20 minutes. Often it is desirable to leave a substance in the
stomach, e.g. after salicylate or iron poisoning, and in that case
lavage is necessary rather than ipecacuanha. Finally ipecacuanha may cause repeated vomiting, and that might cause
danger. Activated charcoal should not be given with ipecacuanha because it prevents it acting as an emetic.

Salt must not be used to cause emesis. It has led to fatalities
as a result of hypernatraemia.

If lavage is to be performed, the child is firmly wrapped in a
blanket, so that his arms are controlled. A tube of a wide bore,
such as 28 FG, should be used. Lavage is not used after a
corrosive substance because of the danger of perforation; and
not after petroleum preparations because of the risk of inhalation, causing pneumonia. Some recommend that activated
charcoal made into a slurry with water should be left in the
stomach for many poisons—such as aspirin, sedative and hyp-
notic drugs.

If children are seen who have taken enteric-coated or other
slow-release tablets, it is important to remember that the
blood levels will be later in rising than with the ordinary type
of tablet. This is particularly important with enteric-coated
aspirin, such as Nuseal or intestinal-release aspirins, such as
Caprin. *If any children are seen having ingested enteric-coated
tablets they must be admitted for at least 48 hours after the initial
evacuation of the stomach and if a child has taken 'slow release'
tablets of any description it is important that this fact is taken
into consideration when they are being admitted, because they
must be admitted for a longer period.*

In cases where children have taken substances with potentially life-threatening effects it is better to arrange admission to
the intensive care unit before these have developed so that
they can be monitored.

It is important to remember that a child who has taken an
overdose of salicylates may have been unwell at the time—so
that there may be an underlying illness requiring treatment.
He may also have been receiving salicylates for some days
before the overdose, so that the serum salicylate level may be

misleading. The dangerously misleading latent period of up to 24 hours or so between the ingestion and the development of symptoms has been mentioned on p. 30. When salicylate poisoning is suspected, the Phenistix test should be applied. Ten per cent ferric chloride added to acid urine gives a purple colour if salicylates have been taken. The serum salicylate level should be determined approximately four hours after the time of the ingestion and the level should be determined again in a further four hours or so but with enteric-coated or sustained-release tablets the *highest level may not be reached before 24 hours or more*. A level above 30–35 mg % (1·9 SI units) is highly dangerous, and overventilation is likely to be a prominent symptom. Methyl salicylate (oil of wintergreen) is particularly dangerous.

It is never too late to evacuate the stomach—even if the aspirin was taken 24 hours before.

Hyperglycaemia is sometimes a feature of salicylate poisoning and may mislead. Hypoglycaemia can also occur but is rare. *In severe aspirin poisoning there is cerebral hypoglycaemia despite normal blood glucose.* If the patient is drowsy or unconscious give glucose intravenously. He may be acidaemic and may deteriorate rapidly.

All children with salicylate intoxication or significant risk of it must be admitted after gastric lavage or emesis. *This must apply in all who have taken methyl salicylate.*

Paracetamol

It is rare to get severe paracetamol poisoning in children because the metabolism in children is different, so they are less likely than adults to get liver damage.

Quantities taken in excess by children are not usually large because the tablets are hard to swallow.

There is a significant lack of correlation between the reported amount ingested and subsequent plasma levels, and hepatic toxicity is usually mild, even with plasma levels commonly lethal in adults.

Other drugs taken at the same time may confuse the diagnosis.

There may be a latent period of up to 48 hours or so between the early nausea and pallor and the development of more serious symptoms.

The stomach should be washed out. If the ingestion was less than ten hours previously (or if in doubt), 1 g of methionine (two capsules), dissolved in 20–30 ml of water, is introduced through the gastric tube. The contents of the capsules take about three minutes to dissolve. Give 1 g of methionine every hour for four hours.

Cysteamine is no longer used. N-acetylcysteine (Parvolex) is widely used in adults. Experience of its use in children is scanty, but it should be available for the rare case when it might be necessary.

Plasma paracetamol levels should be measured about four hours after ingestion and repeated every two to four hours. All cases should be admitted.

Destropropoxyphene and paracetamol (distalgesic)

This can produce respiratory depression and apnoea extremely rapidly and the rapid onset of dextropropoxyphene coma is the major concern.

Intravenous naloxone (Narcan) is extremely urgent. Except in babies, when the initial dose should be reduced, 0·4 mg of naloxone (one ampoule) should be given and further doses intravenously or intramuscularly in two to three minutes.

The effects of the dextropropoxyphene must initially take precedence over the possible effects of the paracetamol.

After initial resuscitation the child must be admitted to intensive care.

Iron

Symptoms may occur early, but more often there is a *latent period of several hours* before serious symptoms develop. The early symptoms are pain, nausea and vomiting, followed by haematemesis; some hours or days later there may be headache, confusion, signs of acute liver failure, convulsions and coma, followed by death.

The treatment is extremely urgent. *Always treat—no matter*

what the parents say about the number of tablets which they think have been ingested.

1 Gastric lavage (intubate before lavage if unconscious). If symptomatic, while preparing the lavage, give 2000 mg of desferrioxamine (Desferal) (four vials) dissolved in 10 ml of water intramuscularly. Lavage with 1% sodium bicarbonate solution or if available a solution of 2000 mg of desferrioxamine dissolved in 1 l of warm water. Leave 5000 mg of desferrioxamine (ten vials) dissolved in 50 ml of water in the stomach.

2 If symptomatic, set up an intravenous drip to give desferrioxamine at 15 mg per kg per hour to a maximum of 80 mg per kg in 24 hours. Add to the usual infusion fluids and *do not give it as an intravenous bolus.*

3 An X-ray of the abdomen after lavage may show the tablets. Send a specimen tablet to the X-ray department. If the tablets are still present give 15 ml of syrup ipecacuanha followed by 200 ml of water.

4 **Admit all cases.**

Diphenoxylate and atropine (Lomotil)

This is an extremely dangerous drug in children. All cases must be admitted for at least 48 hours after lavage or induced emesis. The drug can cause severe respiratory depression and coma. Symptoms may not occur until 36–48 hours after ingestion. Unchanged tablets have been recovered from the stomach 30 hours after ingestion. 0.4 mg of naloxone (Narcan) introduced intravenously should be used for the respiratory depression or coma. The duration of action of naloxone is short and this will need to be repeated intramuscularly in a short time and the child observed carefully for recurrence of symptoms. (Diphenoxylate can be a cause of unexplained abdominal distension in a child. It should never be used in children.)

Alcohol

If the child is conscious the stomach is washed out and glucose is left in. *If he is unconscious the blood sugar is estimated with dextrostix, for there may be severe and very serious hypoglycaemia.* After intravenous glucose consciousness is usually regained. If it is not regained, get an anaesthetist to help with intubation prior to gastric lavage. Admit the child.

In a pre-teen or teenage girl remember the possibility that sexual interference may have occured.

Poisonous plants and berries

Laburnum is the most common cause of poisoning by plants and berries.

Fungi are very difficult for the non-expert to identify. Some of the most dangerous varieties may only produce symptoms about eight hours after ingestion.

In *all* cases, symptomatic or not, there should be immediate evacuation of the stomach by lavage or ipecacuanha and admission for at least 24 hours.

Yew is the most poisonous tree in Britain and can produce convulsions.

Summary

1 Always assume that the child may have taken more than the history suggests. Unless there is incontrovertible evidence to the contrary a mistake about the quantity might be fatal. Keep the original container or tablets.

2 Remember that certain drugs have a dangerous latent period.

3 A good rule is that it is *never* too late to evacuate the stomach after salicylate ingestion.

4 Treat *all* children who may have ingested iron and admit them all.

5 Remember that the child may have some illness other than the results of the ingestion.

6 If parents ring up for advice tell them to bring the container, drugs, etc., with the child.

Further reading

ILLINGWORTH C.M. Childhood poisonings: who is to blame? *Practitioner*, 1974; **213**:73.
ROBERTSON W.O. A further warning on the use of salt as an emetic agent. *J. Pediatr.* 1971; **79**:877.

Coma

A child in coma presents a worrying challenge, particularly if there is no accompanying person who can give a history. The principal causes to consider are as follows:

Head injury (p. 68).
Diabetes mellitus: hyperglycaemia.
Hypoglycaemia.
Effect of drugs, poisons, alcohol, solvent sniffing.
Epilepsy (and an overdose of drugs prescribed for it).
Cerebral haemorrhage, abscess, tumour.
Meningitis, encephalitis.
Hypernatraemia or hyponatraemia: heat stroke, etc.
Liver or kidney failure.
Malaria (if in the tropics or if the child has recently been there).
Sickling.
In the tropics—many acute infections in the presence of malnutrition.
Hysteria.

If there is no sign of head injury, or any other trauma, and no history is available, you will have to rely on the physical examination and special investigations.

Respiratory depression accompanies most forms of profound drug-induced coma. Pinpoint pupils suggest the possibility of the effect of drugs; widely dilated pupils may be due to drugs or to the effect of a convulsion. Unequal pupils may suggest a cerebral lesion on the side of the more dilated pupil. Conjugate deviation of the eyes may suggest irritation on the opposite side of the brain or a destructive lesion on the same side. Nystagmus may be due to antiepileptic drugs or to a posterior fossa lesion. Prick marks on the limbs, or areas of fat atrophy, may give the clue to diabetes. A *mydriatic* (tropicamide or cyclopentolate) *must not be used because it would confuse the diagnosis.*

If there is no sign of injury, and there is no papilloedema or neck stiffness, the smell of acetone in the breath may give the clue to the diagnosis of diabetes: but some doctors have difficulty in smelling acetone.

The *Dextrostix blood sugar estimation should be performed immediately.* If possible a specimen of urine should be obtained. If the blood sugar is low, take blood for electrolytes and the insulin level while the child is still in coma—it will be invaluable for subsequent diagnosis—and treat the hypoglycaemia at once with 20% dextrose intravenously. In cases where intravenous dextrose would be difficult or impossible 1 mg of glucagon (one unit) can be given intramuscularly or subcutaneously, followed by dextrose by mouth as soon as the child is conscious.

Hypoglycaemia

There are many causes of hypoglycaemia other than insulin overdosage. They include:

Starvation—young children rapidly get low blood sugar when they miss meals or are starved too long before an anaesthetic.

Alcohol poisoning (see p. 36).

Rarely—salicylate poisoning, but cerebral hypoglycaemia is common when the child is drowsy.

Chlorpropamide or other antidiabetic drugs; the effect of chlorpropamide (which may have been in use by a parent) is long lasting, and after an apparent 'cure', relapse is liable to occur. The child must be admitted.

Cold injury (newborn, or at any age after exposure) (see p. 55).

Rarely—pancreatic and other tumours, Addison's disease, galactosaemia, glycogenoses, leucine hypersensitivity and Reye's syndrome (liver necrosis with encephalopathy). In Nigeria—cow's urine disease; in Jamaica—ackee fruit poisoning.

Hyperglycaemia

Significant hyperglycaemia (15 mmol [270 mg 100 ml] or more) is nearly always due to diabetes mellitus but it can occur after severe electrolyte disturbance (mainly after gastroenteritis) and serious errors have been made as a result of administrating insulin because of failure to recognize this condition. Hyperglycaemia is a rare complication of salicylate poisoning, Cushing's syndrome, phaeochromocytoma and thyrotoxicosis. It can occur as a transitory phenomenon in the newborn. It is said to occur briefly as a result of severe stress and pain.

The urine should be examined with the Phenistix test for salicylate poisoning, with Clinistix for glucose, and Clinitest for various reducing substances. A high ascorbic acid intake may give a false negative test with Clinistix.

Glycosuria can be caused by a variety of conditions:

Diabetes mellitus

Salicylate poisoning.

Caffeine poisoning.

Renal tubular acidosis, renal glycosuria and nephrotic syndrome.

Transient glycosuria in the newborn (as above).

Dehydration and electrolyte disturbance (as above).

Pituitary disease.

Rarely—fibrocystic disease of the pancreas.

Note that there may be sugar in the urine which was in the bladder before hypoglycaemia developed. There is no significant acidosis or ketosis in the nonketotic hyperosmolar form of diabetic coma.

Take blood for glucose, urea, sodium, potassium, blood gases, haemoglobin, packed cell volume and blood culture. Weigh the child if possible. Insert a nasogastric tube.

The immediate treatment for *diabetic coma* is the administration of 0·9% saline over 30 minutes. Small frequent doses of soluble insulin are now generally used to treat diabetic coma. If a slow infusion pump is available, it is given intravenously at a dose rate of 0·1 unit per kg per hour or if not by giving 0·25 unit per kg intramuscularly. Admit the child forthwith after this emergency treatment.

Coma may be due to a wide variety of drugs. Coma following a fit may be due to the epilepsy or to drugs taken for epilepsy; these may be taken accidentally or on purpose as an overdose.

For poisoning by opium or its analogues, naloxone is the drug of choice and has replaced nalorphine which is a respiratory depressant. It is justifiable to give 0·4 mg of naloxone (Narcan) intravenously or intramuscularly to a child in otherwise unexplained coma with pin-point pupils.

Remember that a child with meningitis may present in coma. If there are any purpuric spots assume it is meningococcal, set up an intravenous line, take blood for culture and give intravenous benzylpenicillin prior to admission. For a one to five-year-old child give 75–150 mg and for a six- to twelve-year-old give 300 mg ($=\frac{1}{2}$ mega unit), dissolved in water and slowly.

Severe drowsiness or coma may result from *hypernatraemia* and from severe dehydration, usually following gastroenteritis. But in the case of young babies hypernatraemia may follow respiratory infections or other cause of fever, if the feeds of dried milk have been overconcentrated. Older, mentally-subnormal children may develop severe dehydration when in an institution, usually following a febrile illness: very high blood urea in such cases may wrongly suggest renal failure.

Whatever the cause of the coma, the first essential is to ensure that there is an airway, and that oxygen is given if necessary.

Treatment of hypoglycaemia is extremely urgent. So too is initiation of treatment in meningococcal infections.

Further reading

CAWTHORNE C.N.H. & HOBDAY J.D. Transient hyperglycaemia, acidosis and coma. *Aust. Paediatr. J.* 1973; **9**:208.

Convulsions

Convulsions are the end-result of a wide variety of causes, and the causes differ with the age of the child.

Newborn

In the *newborn period* the principal causes are as follows:
>   Tetany.
>   Hypoglycaemia.
>   Effect of birth—anoxia, subdural effusion and cerebral haemorrhage.
>   Infection, including tetanus in developing countries.
>   Narcotic withdrawal syndrome.

There are many possible rare metabolic causes.

A convulsion in a newborn baby rarely presents as a major fit. There is usually a mere twitching of a limb or limbs or fluttering of the eyelid; the twitching may migrate from one limb to another. Conjugate deviation of the eyes confirms the diagnosis of a fit. One has to distinguish the tremulousness of a hungry baby; clonic movement of a limb in a fit cannot be stopped by flexing the limb, while jittery, trembling movements can.

Correct diagnosis and treatment are essential. They are more the province of the paediatric in-patient and out-patient department than Casualty but you can investigate the blood glucose and calcium, and treat hypoglycaemia if found. The family doctor can promptly refer the child to hospital for diagnosis and treatment and in the case of hypoglycaemia this is *urgent* to prevent brain damage. It is equally important for doctors to recognize these neonatal convulsions for another reason: they may be due to an infection, which urgently requires treatment.

Infants

In infants after the newborn period, the following are the main causes:

> Febrile convulsions.
> Breath-holding attacks.
> Head injury and subdural effusion (including non-accidental injury).
> Epilepsy.
> Infections, including meningitis, encephalitis and malaria in tropical countries.
> Poisons.
> Dehydration and its repair.

Convulsions are **not** *due to teething.* Febrile convulsions may occur between six months and five years, with only a rapid rise of temperature. There must be a history of the child having been unwell for a few hours before the fit. They are *not focal* in character, do not last more than five to ten minutes and are not repeated (except only a few hours after the first). There is no residual weakness (Todd's paralysis) and there must be no history of fits not conforming with the above criteria. Febrile convulsions are rare before six months. **You must note that any severe major fit causes a rise of temperature, and that fever precipitates fits in epilepsy.**

Breath-holding convulsions ('kinks') are due to the child holding his breath in expiration when thwarted or hurt. These attacks occur between six months and five or six years. The child holds his breath, rapidly goes blue, and if he holds it for a few seconds more he becomes limp; if he holds it a few more seconds he has a major convulsion. Others when hurt have a kind of vasovagal attack and immediately have a fit.

The doctor has to consider the other possibilities: head injury; subdural effusion; infections, especially meningitis; poisoning; and the effect of dehydration, mostly after gastro-enteritis. Hypoglycaemia remains a possibility, even in non-diabetic children; *hence the importance of a blood glucose estimation.*

Many cases of infantile spasms, a form of epilepsy usually starting at four to six months of age and associated with mental subnormality, are due to tuberous sclerosis. The diagnosis can be made in infants by detection of hypopigmented areas on the skin, especially on the trunk, but these may need a Wood's lamp to show them up, and this is out of your province.

All young children brought for a convulsion must be admitted: the serious risk of not doing so lies in particular in the risk of missing an acute pyogenic meningitis. *Children of any age who have had their first fit must be admitted for investigation.* Older children who are already on treatment will usually need admission but if possible you should discuss this with the paediatrician who is already treating them.

Management of a convulsing child

1 Maintain the airway and position appropriately. Give oxygen if necessary.
2 *Do a Dextrostix* and take the temperature. If the

temperature is raised, cool the child by tepid sponging and an electric fan.

3 *Intramuscular paraldehyde* is both effective and safe. The dose is 1 ml per year of age, up to 10 ml. If drawn up and given within a few minutes it can be given in a plastic syringe (it takes 40 minutes for the plunger to begin to deteriorate). The paraldehyde solutions are now much more stable and less likely to give local reactions. It should be given into the upper and outer side of the thigh.

4 *Diazepam.* The strength of *intravenous diazepam* (Valium) is 5 mg per ml. If used this should be with great caution and given *extremely slowly*. There is *a danger not only of respiratory arrest but also of hypotension.* It should *never* be used when there are no facilities for immediate resuscitation but even when there are there may be considerable difficulties following its use. The dose is approximately 1 mg per year of age ($\frac{1}{4}$ mg—$\frac{1}{2}$ mg for young infants) but this must be adjusted according to the size of the child and titrated according to the effect (i.e. stop at once if the convulsion ceases, however little has been given). Intravenous diazepam usually works within a few minutes but *some patients are resistant to diazepam* and you *must not go on giving larger and larger amounts.*

Diazepam can have an irritant effect and should not be given into very small veins.

Although diazepam is used in general practice, because of possible respiratory arrest and hypotension it is risky and paraldehyde is safer. If you are a family doctor send the child to hospital immediately after giving the paraldehyde. Intramuscular diazepam (Valium) is unpredictable in its effects and makes the use of intravenous diazepam subsequently difficult and potentially even more dangerous.

Rectal diazepam is absorbed rapidly from the rectum but the dose cannot be titrated adequately by this method.

5 *Rectal paraldehyde* is absorbed rapidly, is safe and effective, but its use in Casualty may present difficulties if the rectum is not empty.

The solution used is 50% paraldehyde and arachis oil. This is stable for about 14 days. The dose is 0.5 ml per kg of paraldehyde (i.e. 1 ml per kg of enema solution) to a maximum of 30 ml.

The rectum *must* be empty and it is usually necessary to tilt the head down slightly. If retained it is rapidly effective.

6 *If symptoms are not controlled rapidly do not delay in asking for help from the anaesthetist with a thiopentone drip.*

Examine the child thoroughly. Remember that meningococcal septicaemia may present with a fit. If there are any purpuric spots assume it is meningococcal and initiate treatment with intravenous benzylpenicillin. Remember to look inside the lower eyelid for purpura (for one to five-year olds, 75–150 mg, for six to twelve-year olds, 300 mg, dissolved in water and given slowly).

Summary

Children of any age who have had their first fit must be admitted.
Remember to do a Dextrostix—in all ages.
Remember to think of other possible causes, e.g. meningitis, trauma, drugs.
Status epilepticus is an acute emergency requiring immediate treatment.

Further reading

FREEMAN J.M. Neonatal seizures. *J. Pediatr.* 1970; **77**:710.
LIVINGSTON S., BERGMAN W. & PAULI L.L. Febrile convulsions. *Lancet* 1973; **ii**:1441.
VOLPE J. Neonatal seizures. *N. Engl. J. Med.* 1973; **289**:413.

Lacerations

General principles

Much can and must be done to avoid discomfort for the child. Local anaesthetics are of limited use in small children (see p. 15) and one should be more prepared to use general anaesthetics for the purpose of stitching. This applies particularly to many lacerations near the knee. A general anaesthetic may be necessary to clean the wound properly and assess its depth. For traumatic tattoo, the wound should be scrubbed under a general anaesthetic.

Much can be achieved with non-suturing methods, using Ethistrip or Steristrip especially for facial wounds. This does not act as a foreign body, unlike sutures, and so can be left in place several days longer: leave it on the face for at least a week and for seven to ten days on the forehead. Sutures should be used only if essential and if Ethistrip or Steristrip would not be satisfactory.

Wherever possible use non-stick dressings, such as Melolin, because it will be much less uncomfortable to remove later; but it must not be used for infected wounds.

Avoid frequent dressing of wounds. Wounds over the knee, however, should be inspected 48 hours after suture. Most other wounds need be seen only when the sutures are removed. The removal of adherent dressings is not only painful for the child, but it actively delays healing by pulling the top off the wound. Doctors must resist the temptation to keep looking at the wound to see if it is healing.

Wherever possible, put injured parts at rest. Where there is laceration near a joint, the limb should be immobilized. All children with wounds over the knee which require suturing should be prevented from weight bearing for 48 hours. If the wound is deep or extensive, the knee should be splinted in 15° of flexion. For wounds around the ankle a back splint should be applied. For wounds around the elbow, a collar and cuff sling is adequate.

Avoid prophylactic antibiotics (see p. 13) but take swabs from infected wounds in order to determine the sensitivity in

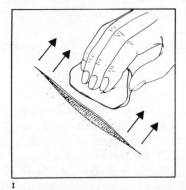 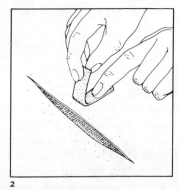

1 2

Fig. 1 Clean and dry the skin for at least three inches around the wound, working from the wound edges outward.

Fig. 2 Starting from the middle of the wound, apply half of the strip to one **dried** wound margin and press firmly into place.

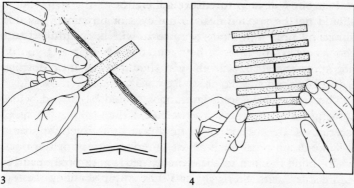

3   4

Fig. 3 Using finger pressure or forceps, draw the skin together, achieving a slightly everted edge. Press the free half of the strip firmly into place.

Fig. 4 As in suturing, space out the strips carefully to allow the wound to breathe. Do not completely occlude the wound.

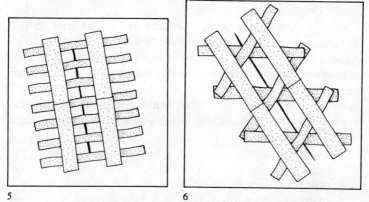

5   6

Fig. 5 The closure strips may be given extra support by placing broader strips parallel to the wound.

Fig. 6 For wounds over joints a criss-cross application gives greater security.

case antibiotic treatment is necessary. For haemolytic streptococcal infections, give penicillin for a full ten days.

Specific instructions

The method of applying Ethistrip or Steristrip is shown in Figs 1–6. First clean the skin thoroughly and dry it. Tincture of benzoin will help to ensure adherence of the strip, but it should not be applied near to the eyes or on superficial skin abrasions near a wound, because it will be painful. There should always be a space between adhesive strips. If you do not apply the strip yourself, you should check their position before the child goes home.

The area around scalp lacerations should be shaved before suturing. Do not apply a dressing to the scalp or to facial lacerations. Do not apply 'plastic sprays' or antibiotic sprays.

Wounds on areas such as the anterior surface of the tibia, where bone is close to the surface, need more prolonged reinforcement with Steristrip or Ethistrip for about two weeks after the sutures have been removed at ten days; otherwise they are liable to break down.

Have an X-ray taken for all but trivial or superficial wounds around the knee, and for all lacerations including eye injuries caused by glass (glass is radio-opaque).

A child with a deep or dirty wound around the knee should be admitted for surgical debridement under a general anaesthetic.

Remove sutures from the face and scalp at five days, from the arms, chest and abdomen at seven days, and from the back and legs at ten to fourteen days. When Steristrip or Ethistrip is used they must be left in place considerably longer than sutures in the same area.

It is rarely necessary to suture a lacerated tongue—even the most ragged looking lacerations heal well. The main indication for suture is uncontrollable bleeding.

In small children when there is a laceration of the lip, as long as the red margins are properly approximated, and provided that the laceration is at right angles to the edge of the lip, it will heal without any further sutures in the lip itself being necessary, and will give a good scar which matches the vertical lines naturally present on the lips.

Foreign bodies

The casualty doctor and family doctor have constantly to remember the possibility that a child's symptoms may be due to a foreign body. It is by no means always the case that the history obtained will give any inkling that a foreign body was inhaled, ingested or otherwise introduced. For instance, in an Australian study of over 230 inhaled foreign bodies, there was a history of inhalation of the foreign body in only one-third (Pyman 1971). Awareness of the possibility in many different situations will increase the likelihood that one will obtain a history of possible introduction of a foreign body. *If a mother herself suspects the possibility, however unlikely the story seems, you must take her suspicions seriously and investigate.* The subject is an important one: it is said that in the USA there are 2900 deaths each year from inhaled or ingested foreign bodies (Majd *et al.* 1977).

The ear

A foreign body in the ear is not an emergency. Sometimes the foreign body is readily accessible to forceps—but one must guard against the risk of pushing it farther into the canal or damaging the drum by it or by the forceps. In most cases gentle syringing is successful and much safer for the relatively inexperienced. Do not attempt to syringe if the whole external meatus is blocked or if the object is paper or vegetable matter because it would swell up.

After removing the foreign body examine the ear to ensure that there is not a second object left behind, and that no damage has been done by the foreign body. It is far better to ask the ear, nose and throat surgeon to remove the foreign body in his next out-patient session or at the end of an operating list than to risk damage to the ear drum, which may happen, especially in a young, unco-operative child.

The nose

A foreign body in the nose is not an emergency. The common complaint is that there is an offensive, purulent nasal discharge, usually unilateral—but sometimes bilateral if there is an object in each nostril.

Sometimes the object can be gently milked out of the nose

by pressure above it. If a child is old enough, he should be asked to blow while one applies pressure to occlude the other side of the nose. If you can see the object, apply pressure behind it so that he does not sniff and draw it further in. It may be possible to get a bent ring probe along the septum past the foreign body and behind it or to get hold of it with nasal forceps so that it can be brought down. If you can get hold of the foreign body, remember that the entrance to the nostrils is the narrowest part so put your finger behind it on the nose while extracting it or it may disappear from sight again.

If you think you may have difficulty or if the child is young and unco-operative do not try to remove the foreign body but ask the ear, nose and throat surgeon to deal with it either in the next out-patient session or at the end of an operating list.

The eye

Many foreign bodies can be removed by gentle irrigation with saline. If the foreign body can be seen and irrigation does not remove it, anaesthetize the eye with 1% Amethocaine and gently remove it with an eye spud or with the top of a needle attached to an empty syringe. The syringe gives more control over the needle. Any embedded foreign bodies *must be referred to an eye surgeon*. If there is a suspected foreign body under the upper lid, the lid should be everted by applying a match stick across the base of the tarsal plate and everting the lid by means of the eye lashes. If it is thought that the cornea may have been damaged, a drop of fluorescein will show whether it has been scratched. It may be wise also to insert two or three drops of chloramphenicol if it is thought that the cornea has been scratched. If amethocaine anaesthetic has been used a pad must be placed over the eye when the child leaves, keeping the pad in place for 24 hours. If the eye may have been damaged by glass, the eye specialist should be asked to see the eye with the help of a slip lamp. If there is any possibility of a foreign body being metal or glass, an X-ray must be taken. Remember to make sure that the child has been immunized against tetanus (p. 14).

The throat and tonsils

Children are often brought because the parents think that a bone or toothbrush bristle has become stuck in the throat. The area in which they are most likely to be found is at the lower pole of the tonsil and you should look carefully here. Often the complaint of soreness is the result of a minor scratch by something like a fish-bone so that it is reasonable to re-examine the child in half to one hour. If the symptoms persist and nothing can be seen on examination, ask the ear, nose and throat surgeon for help. If the object is farther down the throat, the ear, nose and throat specialist should be asked to see the child without delay. X-ray examination should be done but may not be helpful in reaching a diagnosis.

Inhaled foreign body

An object may be inhaled by a child because he was running about or laughing with food in his mouth, was throwing peanuts into the air and catching them with an open mouth, was holding an object (such as a pin or hairclip) in his mouth, or for other reasons. Contrary to common belief, *rubber objects often show in an X-ray.*

Larynx

A foreign body in the larynx is an emergency. It may cause cough, stridor, cyanosis, choking, hoarseness or aphonia. As an immediate measure, the child is held upside down and his back is slapped. If that fails, he should be taken to hospital immediately; if in the casualty department, the ear, nose and throat specialist should be asked to see the child.

Be prepared, if necessary, while arrangements are being made for a bracheostomy to stick a large needle such as a lumbar puncture needle through the crico-thyroid membrane to relieve acute airway obstruction which would not be helped by intubation. Cricothyreotomy cannulae are available for this purpose.

Trachea

A foreign body in the trachea may cause wheezing, dyspnoea and a rattling noise on respiration. The child should be seen forthwith by the ear, nose and throat specialist and admitted.

Bronchi

Nuts, peas and other vegetable matter, coins, pins and other objects may be inhaled. It is important to realize that though there may be the story of a sudden cough with dyspnoea, *there is often no cough at all*. In 40% of Pyman's series there was a wheeze but no cough. One should suspect the presence of a foreign body when a non-asthmatic child develops a wheeze, and there is no response to bronchodilators. The child's developmental age is relevant. Under the age of six months he is unlikely to pick up a small enough object and take it to the mouth; he is more likely to do so when he develops finger–thumb apposition (at ten months) and begins to creep and get around. The common story is that of an attack of coughing, followed by a latent period of days or weeks, followed then by symptoms and signs of a complication. The signs then may be those of pneumonia, emphysema, atelectasis and displacement of the trachea or apex beat: but often there are no abnormal physical signs at all.

It is important that nuts, peas and other vegetable matter should be removed promptly, because they swell up in the presence of secretions. As a first-aid measure, it is a mistake to invert the child or to try to make him sick: the object may become impacted in the larynx.

The X-ray of the chest may be normal: *it is a common mistake to assume that a normal X-ray excludes a foreign body*. Crayon or plastic material is usually not radio-opaque. Diagnosis has to be established by bronchoscopy.

It is important that a bronchoscopy is done as *early as possible* because it is infinitely wiser to have one done early than to wait for complications. *Do not hesitate to ask a thoracic surgeon or an ear, nose and throat surgeon to see any child with a suggestive history*.

Other foreign bodies

The oesophagus

Ingested foreign bodies especially include hairclips, coins, safety-pins and a variety of toys. They present an emergency if they become impacted in the cervical area or cause obstruction anywhere. The usual three sites for impaction are the level of the fourth cervical vertebra, the aortic arch and the diaphragm. As in the case of foreign bodies in the bronchus, there may be three phases: coughing and choking at first, followed by a latent period, and then by the results of complications, including pulmonary symptoms.

An older child can localize the site of obstruction and there may also be retching and salivation if the obstruction is high up. Many objects are radio-opaque. Remember that rubber may also show up on X-ray.

In most cases the object has to be removed. Some will observe a child for a maximum of 12 hours if the impacted object is a round one. In any case the child should be admitted.

No emetics should be given in an effort to retrieve it by vomiting.

Stomach

There is a dangerous tendency to take the presence of a foreign body in the stomach too lightly and to assume that it will pass safely. It is true that 80–90% of foreign bodies reaching the stomach will pass without trouble but the remainder do not. It depends partly on the shape of the object and its size in relation to that of the child. Hairclips and open safety-pins should usually be removed. They are apt to become impacted at the duodenal junction or the ileocaecal area. The child should be admitted for observation. The average time taken by an object to pass through the alimentary tract is five or six days but it is reasonable to observe a round object in the stomach for up to two to three weeks; then discuss possible removal with the surgeons. X-rays should not be taken more often than every seven days because of the irradiation involved. The parents should be told not to alter the diet, by giving extra roughage, and not to give a purgative. They should be told to examine the stools to attempt to detect the passage of the object: but it is common that they do not see it even though it is passed. If there is any vomiting, pain or fever the parents should be told to return at once and the child should be referred immediately to the surgeons.

Bladder

Safety-pins and other objects may be pushed into the bladder and cause haematuria.

Vagina

A wide variety of foreign bodies have been introduced into the vagina. The usual complaint is a purulent vaginal discharge. The child should be referred to a paediatric surgeon or gynaecologist.

The skin

No attempt should be made in a doctor's surgery or casualty department to remove foreign bodies such as needles or glass in the hands and feet unless they are clearly visible or palpable immediately under the skin. Any others causing symptoms should be dealt with in a clean theatre by a surgeon who has ensured a bloodless field.

Many small foreign bodies will gradually work to the surface if left and may be easy to remove later: but before knowingly leaving them it would be wise to obtain an expert opinion.

When a hand or foot has been cut by glass, an X-ray should be taken to detect residual glass particles.

Summary

1 Sites where removal is urgent are:
  Larynx
  Trachea.
  Oesophagus.
  Chest.

2 Do *not* attempt to remove foreign bodies in the hands, feet, etc., unless you can see them or feel them immediately under the skin.

3 Remember that glass usually shows up on X-rays and *any* wound which has involved glass must be X-rayed. Rubber (especially if coloured) often shows up on X-ray.

4 Do *not* give emetics for swallowed and impacted foreign bodies.

5 A normal chest X-ray *does not* exclude an inhaled foreign body.

Further reading

MAJD N.S., MOFENSON H.C. & GREENSHER J. Lower airway foreign body aspiration in children. *Clin. Pediatr. Phila.* 1977; **16**:13.
PYMAN C. Inhaled foreign bodies in children. A review of 230 cases. *Med. J. Aust.* 1971; **1**:62.

Burns and scalds

Much of what I wrote in the section on non-accidental injury on the importance of the history (see p. 17) applies equally here. One must remember the possibility that the burn was due to child abuse. It is important to record exactly how the burn was acquired, the exact time at which it occurred, and the time at which the child arrived at the casualty department or doctor's surgery.

The general condition of the child must be recorded, with particular regard to his colour, restlessness, pulse, and respiration rate: if he has been exposed to smoke (as in a burning house) his voice must be noted, with the appearance of the pharynx. The percentage of burnt area is estimated as shown in Fig. 7.

All children with anything but the most trivial burns must be admitted: these include all children with electrical burns, burns of the genitalia, buttocks or perineum, and all with any but small trivial burns of the hands and face. Any burns which are circumferential, that is involving both sides of a limb, must be admitted. The child with burns near to the eyes must be admitted and seen by the ophthalmologist. Electrical burns nearly always cause deep tissue damage. The doctor should

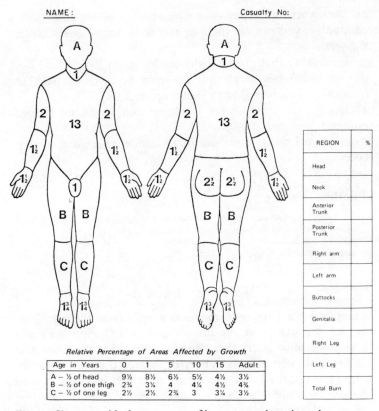

REGION	%
Head	
Neck	
Anterior Trunk	
Posterior Trunk	
Right arm	
Left arm	
Buttocks	
Genitalia	
Right Leg	
Left Leg	
Total Burn	

Relative Percentage of Areas Affected by Growth

Age in Years	0	1	5	10	15	Adult
A – ½ of head	9½	8½	6½	5½	4½	3½
B – ½ of one thigh	2¾	3¼	4	4¼	4½	4¾
C – ½ of one leg	2½	2½	2¾	3	3¼	3½

Fig. 7 Chart to enable the percentage of burnt area to be estimated.

know that a severe electric shock (e.g. due to contacting a power cable) may be associated with dislocation of the shoulder. A child who was in a burning house, *even though there is no evidence of burning of the skin*, must be admitted *immediately* to the intensive care unit, particularly if he is wheezing: this is because of injury to the respiratory passages by fumes.

Special investigations required are the haemoglobin, haematocrit, electrolytes, blood urea and bicarbonate, serum proteins and blood for cross-matching. The fluid intake and output is charted. The child's weight is determined or estimated.

If the area burnt approaches 10%, intravenous plasma is required; the quantity to be given in the *first* four *hours* after the injury in ml is:

$$\frac{\text{percentage of burn} \times \text{weight in kg}}{2}$$

Haemaccel (Hoechst), which is a plasma substitute, in the form of a 3·5% colloidal infusion solution, with a molecular weight of 35 000, can be used instead of plasma. Sedation is not given as a routine. There must be an adequate airway and oxygen may be indicated. Adherent clothes, unless chemicals are involved, are not removed before admission to the ward.

For any but the most trivial burns the plastic surgeon or burns unit is consulted. Opinions differ as to the management of a trivial burn, as to whether the blister should be removed or not but with a simple dressing of Jelonet or Bactigras which is *left in place for at least a week* the majority heal without trouble.

Over the dressing a thick layer of gamgee is placed to absorb oozing: this can be changed if necessary without disturbing the dressing which is in contact with the burn itself.

Remember that tetanus can be a risk following burns.

The mother should be told that it is important that the child with a burn or scald who is allowed home should drink plenty of fluid.

Further reading

HARRIS F. *Paediatric Fluid Therapy*. Oxford: Blackwell Scientific Publications, 1972.

Heat-stroke

Heat exhaustion occurs in hot weather when insufficient water and salt has been taken to replace the loss in sweat. The child who is irritable, complaining of dizzyness, headache and feeling sick, soon recovers when put into a cool place and given cool drinks.

It is dangerous when this stage is passed, particularly if the sweating mechanism fails so that the core temperature rises rapidly. The rectal temperature may reach 43° or 45°C and consciousness is lost. At that stage the skin is usually hot and dry. This is heat-stroke.

Heat-stroke may develop if dehydration due to sweating has been severe, so that sweating ceases; if the skin is covered extensively with oily or greasy preparations; or if there has been a period of fasting or insufficient fluid intake before hard physical exercise in a hot climate.

Children with cystic fibrosis are at great risk. Drugs such as atropine, the phenothiazine derivatives, tricyclic antidepressants, monoamine oxidase inhibitors, and amphetamine can precipitate heat-stroke. In addition, malignant hyperthermia can occur under general anaesthesia when a drug such as halothane is used. Some families with differing myopathies are particularly prone to this type of heat-stroke. A combination of extreme physical exercise in hot weather with ingestion of a drug such as amphetamine is dangerous. The diagnosis may be difficult and the differential diagnoses include epilepsy, meningitis, encephalitis, and in some countries malaria.

Suspect heat-stroke if a child loses consciousness in conditions of extreme heat after exercise. The skin will not be dry in all cases. Measure the rectal temperature. Rapid cooling is essential. The skin is kept wet, and cool air played over it, or the child is wrapped in a cool, wet sheet or put into a cold bath until the rectal temperature reaches 39°C. Fluid and electrolyte imbalance has to be corrected.

The child is admitted to the intensive care unit.

He may develop renal failure, severe cerebral effects and disturbances of the clotting mechanism.

If he survives there may be renal damage and he may be left with permanent serious cerebral sequelae.

Further reading

SHIBOLET S., LANCASTER M.C. & DANON Y. Heat-stroke—a review. *Aviation Space and Environmental Medicine* 1976; **47**:280.

Cold injury

(See also the next section on drowning and immersion hypothermia.)

Cold injury can occur at any age after exposure to cold: it is important in the newborn period because the diagnosis can readily be missed. The symptoms and signs are lethargy, loss of appetite, slow feeding, a red face and extremities, in most cases with oedema of hands and feet and a cold skin. There may be oliguria, haematemesis and melaena. The child, at least in the earlier stages, does not look ill. The diagnosis is made by a low-reading thermometer (measuring 24–41°C).

The usual practice is to resist all temptation to warm the child rapidly. He is allowed to warm up slowly and spontaneously in a room having a temperature of 18–24°C, fully clothed, without additional external heat. Some advocate a 15% to 20% glucose drip into the stomach; some also give an antibiotic because hypothermia may result from an infection, but it is not usually necessary. Only if the temperature is below 30°C should immediate warming methods be used, because otherwise there is a danger of ventricular fibrillation. If the temperature is below 30°C, he is placed in a warm bath at 44°C or as hot as the hand can stand. As soon as the temperature rises above 30°C, he is dried and rewarmed slowly without actual heat. The dangers of rapid warming are ventricular fibrillation, acidosis and hypoglycaemia with fits.

Any baby or young child who is lethargic with loss of appetite should be seen by a paediatrician and admitted.

Further reading

BOWER B.D., JONES L.F. & WEEKS M.M. Cold injury in the new-born. *Br. Med. J.* 1960; i:303.

DRUG AND THERAPEUTICS BULLETIN Emergency treatment of accidental hypothermia 1971; 9:6.

MANN T.P. Neonatal cold injury. *Lancet* 1957; i:229.

Drowning and immersion hypothermia

Many patients brought in after rescue from water die not of drowning but of hypothermia.

Hypothermia is particularly likely to be the main problem when the body is in a life-jacket and recovered apparently dead. Hypothermia is of particular importance because, if it is not recognized, the child who is recovered flaccid, with fixed dilated pupils, 'pulseless', and with a flat ECG may be regarded as dead and no efforts made to resuscitate him. *The only way in which a diagnosis of death from hypothermia can be made is failure to respond to correct resuscitation.*

Below a core temperature of 30°C, consciousness is usually lost. A rectal temperature is the most useful one but the diagnosis is mainly clinical. If the child is conscious or semi-conscious he is unlikely to die of hypothermia but there is a dangerous period after rescue when as a result of cold blood returning from the limbs, the core temperature may drop further so that insulation of the patient and re-warming is urgent.

'Space blankets' are no more effective than polythene bags but fibre-pile exposure bags (Eskimos) made by Vista of Glossop and designed primarily for mountain rescue can be valuable. As soon as possible the child should be immersed in a bath (with water as hot as the hand can bear, 40–44°C).

Anoxia and inhalation are the other main problems in the near-drowned child.

Debris or vomit can obstruct the airways. Inhalation of fresh water into the lungs causes haemodilution, a fall in blood sodium and chloride and occasionally some haemolysis.

Inhalation of salt water causes hypernatraemia and haemo-concentration. It is thought that in very cold water there is a more intense response similar to the 'diving reflex' which occurs in diving mammals, in which there is shut-down of the peripheral circulation but preservation of circulation to the brain and heart. There is a profound bradycardia and to some extent the lungs are protected against the water by spasm of the glottis. This reflex is well developed in small children. In addition their large body surface in relation to their weight means that their core temperature will fall rapidly and be a protective mechanism against cerebral damage.

Even if the child is apparently dead and without a palpable pulse prolonged efforts must be made to resuscitate him. These must be continued until circulation and respiration are re-established or brain death has occurred. While resuscitation is continued the child must be rewarmed so that the core temperature is 30°C. Below that the diagnosis of brain death is impossible. Efforts at resuscitation may last for up to two hours.

If the circulation and ventilation becomes adequate, the child is transferred to the intensive care unit for long-term management. The prognosis of the 'nearly drowned' depends on the level of consciousness one or two hours after rescue. Three groups are recognized:

a   Awake.

b   Blunted consciousness but rousable and normal response to pain.

c   Comatose, abnormal response to pain and abnormal respiration.

The most serious subdivision of group C is when the child is flaccid and shows no response to pain.

Ordinary medical management should result in the recovery of children in groups A and B.

In the comatose group it is now thought that the raised intracranial pressure due to later brain swelling affects the outlook greatly and that neurones which have survived the original injury may be damaged. The time at which raised intracranial pressure occurs is earlier with the severest injuries but the time is variable.

The problems which have to be dealt with in the intensive care unit are: hyperhydration (with cerebral oedema) following ingestion or aspiration of water as well as of any fluids given during attempts at resuscitation; the effects on the lungs of water or foreign material; and the fact that after near-drowning there is usually a rise of temperature which can have serious effects on the brain.

Once the circulation is stable, fluid is restricted to one-third of maintenance requirements and active measures are taken to reduce cerebral oedema. The child's body temperature is maintained as near to 30°C as possible to reduce cerebral oxygen requirements, but it should not fall below 28°C because ventricular fibrillation may then occur.

If a child is brought in apparently dead through drowning remember the possibility of hypothermia and that in this condition the only certain way of diagnosing death is failure to respond to prolonged resuscitation and rewarming.

Further reading

CONN A.W. *et al.* Cerebral resuscitation in near-drowning. *Paed. Clinics N. Am.* 1979; **26**(3):691.

KEATINGE W.R. *Survival in Cold Water.* Oxford: Blackwell Scientific Publications, 1969.

MODELL J.H. *et al.* Near-drowning; correlation of level of consciousness and survival. *Canad. anaesth. Soc. J.* 1980; **27**(3):211.

Cardiac and respiratory arrest

In children, arrest from primary cardiac causes is rare. Most will have primary respiratory arrest, with cardiac arrest following because of hypoxia. Important causes include foreign bodies, poisoning and infection. *The airway and adequate ventilation are thus particularly important.*

Get someone to summon skilled help, but meanwhile *clear the mouth*—by suction if possible, or manually insert an airway and give 100% oxygen.

In almost all children adequate ventilation can be obtained with a self-inflating bag and mask and time should not be wasted in trying to intubate the child unless the operator is competent to do so.

Oesophageal obturator airways, which are extremely useful in adults, are not yet available for children but are being developed.

Check the movement of the chest wall. Ventilation must be gentle—just enough to make the chest rise. The rate in infants should be 20 per minute and in children 15 per minute.

After four breaths with an open airway determine whether cardiac arrest has also occurred—feel the pulse over the carotid, femoral or brachial artery (on the inside of the upper arm mid-way between the shoulder and elbow). *If there is no pulse begin external cardiac massage at once.*

For a baby the thumbs are brought together over the mid-sternum, with the hands round the thorax, and pressure is applied by the thumbs approximately 90 times a minute, relaxing the hands between compression.

In young children the heart is compressed with the heel of the hand over the mid-sternum at 60–80 times per minute. The ratio of compression to respiration is 5 : 1. Each compression should give a palpable pulse. When ventilation is adequate and someone is available, attach an ECG monitor and insert an intravenous line percutaneously or by cut-down. If there is asystole give 0·1 ml per kg of 1 in 10 000 adrenaline intravenously or, if necessary, into the heart. For an intracardiac injection insert a long needle just below and medial to the left nipple, directing the tip posteriorly towards the spine.

Sodium bicarbonate may be necessary because of the metabolic acidosis which results from cardiac arrest, but be *extremely cautious* about giving it in children. Give 1 ml per kg of 8·4% (i.e. 1 mEq per kg) slowly if hypoxia has been prolonged. It is highly irritant and small peripheral veins should not be used. (1 mEq = 1·6 ml of 5% solution of sodium bicarbonate, 1 mEq = 2·0 ml of 4·2% and 1 mEq = 1·0 ml of 8·4%.)

The ECG will be needed to monitor further drug therapy. If *ventricular fibrillation* occurs defibrillation will be needed. The shocks given *must* be related to the age of the child—20 J for infants, 75 J for children.

Begin cardiac massage immediately. If unsuccessful give adrenaline and a further shock.

Endotracheal intubation

A laryngoscope with a curved blade is useless under the age of six months; the tongue is too big and the epiglottis is too flaccid. A straight 'infant' model is needed. It is pushed right back almost into the oesophagus and then withdrawn slowly so that the epiglottis is on the far side of the laryngoscope blade, away from the operator. When a curved blade is used in the older child the epiglottis is on the *near* side of the laryngoscope, nearer to the operator.

As a rough guide the endotracheal tube should be the same size as the child's external nares or the diameter of the tip of the little finger (Table 1). In length it should be twice the distance from the side of the nose to the front of the ear.

Table 1 Approximate size of endotracheal tubes.

Age	Magill	Internal diameter (mm)
6 months	000 or 00	3·0–3·5
6 months–1 year	0	4·0
1–2 years	1	4·5
2–6 years	2 or 3	5·0 and 5·5
6–8 years	4	6·0
8–10 years	5	6·5
10–14 years	6 or 7	7·0 and 7·5

Fix the tube immediately with:

1   A strip of zinc oxide strapping across the tube and the upper lip.

2   A strip across the forehead holding the extension tubes.

3   A strip from the chin holding the mouth shut and going right over the nose to the forehead (see Fig. 8).

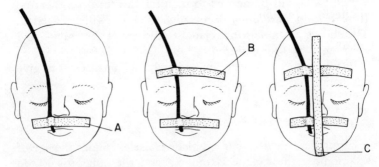

Fig. 8 Method of holding an endotracheal tube in place. (A) A strip across the upper lip holding the endotracheal tube. (B) A strip across the forehead. (C) A strip from the chin over the nose to the forehead holding the mouth shut.

Acute heart failure

If treatment is urgent prior to admission, give half the digitalizing dose. The total digitalizing dose would be 0·03 mg per kg of digozin. The child is then admitted.

Severe acute asthma

Every attempt is made to calm the child by talking to him. Nebulized salbutamol is extremely useful in an acute attack and many children are now used to it. The great virtue is that the method is simple, can be started rapidly and is painless. It is unlikely to be effective in very young children, under the age of 18–20 months, but even in these it is worth trying.

There are different types of nebulizers and· you should become familiar with the model available. The nebulizer solution of salbutamol (Ventolin) is 0·5%. The dosage for a child under five years old is 0·5 ml which equals 2·5 mg of salbutamol; that for a child over five years old is 1·0 ml which equals 5·0 mg of salbutamol. This is made up with 2·0 ml of normal saline. It can be given by mouthpiece or with a mask in younger children.

The pulse should be checked before and after it is given. It normally takes five to seven minutes to give the nebulized solution. The increase in peak flow occurs in about ten minutes.

If the child's condition does not improve sufficiently for him to be allowed home, he will have to be admitted, so that it is extremely unlikely that a second dose of nebulized salbutamol will be given in Casualty. Provided that the child has received the whole amount (because if not it may be repeated earlier) the frequency of repetition is after about three to four hours.

Severe attacks which do not respond to nebulized salbutamol need other drugs. Subcutaneous adrenaline is effective (0·2–0·3 ml of 1 in 1000 solution) but has largely been replaced by terbutaline (Bricanyl). This should not be used in combination with aminophylline or related compounds.

Table 2 Dosage of terbutaline (Bricanyl).

Weight of child (kg)	Dosage (mg subcutaneously)
12–20	0·10
20–30	0·15
30–40	0·20
40–50	0·25

50–100 mg of intravenous hydrocortisone may be given. It is essential to ensure that hydration is adequate. In a severe attack intravenous fluids are required and 0·18% saline in 4·8% dextrose should be given.

Terbutaline contains 0·5 mg (500 μg) in 1 ml of saline solution. The amount given is as shown in Table 2.

Remember that a sudden deterioration may be due to a pneumothorax (see p. 75) and that in an unexpectedly severe attack in an asthmatic child the possibility of an inhaled foreign body should be considered. A child with severe, acute asthma should be admitted to the intensive care unit because the help of anaesthetists may be necessary.

For other causes of wheezing see p. 139.

Anaphylaxis

If the anaphylaxis is due to an injection into a limb, obstruct the venous return by a tourniquet proximal to the injection site for not more than ten minutes; but *do not forget it is on. Give adrenaline—intramuscularly as quickly as possible.* Repeat the dose in ten minutes if necessary. The dosage for a child of less than one year old is 0·05 ml of 1 in 1000 solution; for a child one to five years old 0·1–0·4 ml; six to twelve years old 0·5 ml; and twelve years old and over 0·5–0·75 ml. Adrenaline can also be injected around the site of the injection.

Oxygen should be given early because the hypoxaemia which results from oedema of the airways is dangerous.

If the child does not improve rapidly, set up a rapid intravenous infusion of saline or other plasma volume expander.

The *urgent* treatment is that listed above.

Hydrocortisone succinate (100 mg) should then be given intravenously.

1 mg per kg of diphenhydramine intramuscularly (maximum 50 mg) may also be useful.

Acute anaphylaxis should be minimized by taking a proper history of any known sensitivity, e.g. to penicillin, *before* it is given.

Road-traffic accidents

(See also the sections on injuries to the head, facial bones, thorax and abdomen, pp. 68–77.)

As with other accidents, one must determine the exact nature of the accident, how it happened, the exact time at which it occurred, and the condition of the child immediately after (in respect of concussion).

The whole child must be examined, fully undressed, before X-ray examination. *The time of the examination should be recorded,* and *all the findings, positive or negative.* It is particularly important for medico-legal purposes that a note should be made about all parts examined. The size and equality of the pupils, the pulse, respiration rate, colour and blood pressure are noted, and also the child's level of responsiveness. Any changes in the child's condition and the clinical findings which are noted when the child is re-examined are recorded as is the *time.*

For notes about limb X-rays, see p. 85. For abdominal injuries ask for erect and supine positions if possible, and look for air under the diaphragm as an indicator of perforation of the alimentary tract. If an erect view is impossible, a lateral decubitus position is requested. The urine is examined for blood, albumin and sugar.

The possibility of referred pain must be remembered (p. 11) and the highly important fact that a fracture in one site (e.g. the tibia) may cause an apparent suppression of pain at another damaged site (e.g. the hip). *If a child with head injury shows significant shock, one should look elsewhere for the cause such as a ruptured spleen, or haemorrhage from a pleural or peritoneal injury.* The possibility of a *cervical injury is easily forgotten.*

Treatment

In the case of a seriously injured child, after a rapid initial
assessment the first essential is to give oxygen, having established an airway by suction and intubation if necessary (see the
section on cardiac and respiratory arrest, p. 62). Pass a nasogastric tube, take blood for cross-matching and set up an intravenous infusion of plasma or plasma substitute, e.g. Haemaccel.

*A shocked child has lost at least a quarter of his normal blood
volume and you should assume that an injured child is shocked if
his blood pressure is below 70 mm per Hg and he has pale extremities and tachycardia.* Give an initial bolus of 20 ml per kg of
plasma or plasma substitute (e.g. Haemaccel). 0·9% saline is
not physiological in children and should only be used as an
expander if plasma is unavailable. If the child stays hypoten-
sive with a raised pulse give a further bolus.

The upper limits of a normal pulse are 160 per minute in
infants, 140 per minute below the age of five years and 120 per
minute above.

A rough guide to the normal systolic blood-pressure in
children is 80 plus twice the age in years.

If it is reasonably possible, because the situation is less
acute, the intravenous infusion is postponed, for reasons of
convenience, until necessary X-rays have been taken, but this
is not possible in the case of an acute emergency. Sedatives
should not be given if there is a possibility of an intra-
abdominal injury, or if it would render the assessment of the
level of consciousness more difficult. An injection of tetanus
toxoid is given before the child leaves the casualty department
if he has not had a booster or completed immunization in the
last three years.

Head injury
The history

Data needed include *the exact nature of the accident*, the exact
time at which it occurred, the cause of the accident and how it
happened, and in particular *the condition* of the *child before and*

after the accident. One must also determine whether there were any circumstances to suggest the possibility of non-accidental injury.

The condition of the child *before* the accident may be important, for he may have been unwell. Subsequently, when he is unwell after the accident, he is taken to the doctor who may assume that his symptoms are due to the accident, when in fact they are due to an infection such as otitis media or urinary tract infection. *It is particularly important to know whether the child has previously had convulsions, for the accident may have been the result of a fit.* One must also know whether there are any other relevant defects, such as a blood disease. One should ask whether the child was receiving drugs for any purpose before the accident: they may have been partly responsible for it.

It is then essential to determine what the child was like immediately after the accident, with particular regard to whether he was fully conscious, knew what had happened (and was therefore not concussed), was drowsy, vomited, had a headache, was speaking normally, had no double vision (which would suggest an occipital injury), was unsteady, or whether there was bleeding from the nose or ears (suggesting the possibility of a skull fracture). It is useful to know whether he cried immediately after the accident (and was therefore conscious). The history as always, is taken *before* the examination, while a nurse is recording pulse, blood pressure, etc., and *before* special investigations such as an X-ray are requested, *but you must have seen the child and made sure that no immediate resuscitation is required.*

The examination

The child should not be given a sedative, nor should a mydriatic be used to dilate the pupils, because either would confuse the diagnosis. The exact *time* of the examination is recorded. Though obviously one is particularly concerned with the examination of the head and the nervous system, the whole child must be examined, the child being fully undressed. There may be a coexisting and fairly relevant medical disease.

There may be injuries elsewhere. *If the child is in a state of shock, one must look for a cause elsewhere, such as an abdominal injury* (p. 76). The blood pressure, pulse and respiration rate and limb movements are noted. Many hospitals use observation charts based on the Glasgow coma-scale record-system and if possible these should be used for any child in whom consciousness is or may be impaired. This will include not only children with head injuries but children with poisoning, etc.

Where relevant, serial examinations are made in an observation room to record the pulse, respiration rate, blood pressure, and changes in state of consciousness and responsiveness, *recording the time of each examination. Changes in the state* of the child are vital in determining whether the child is improving or deteriorating. Serial clinical assessments are likely to be much more useful than an X-ray of the skull.

The examination of the head includes inspection of the nose and ears for escape of blood or cerebrospinal fluid, suggesting a fractured skull. If clear fluid drips from the nose, differentiate CSF from nasal secretion by using Clinistix to detect glucose in the fluid. Palpate the fontanelle and the sutures (in the case of a baby) for signs of increased intracranial pressure. Inspect for facial or other bruising, for scars and burns, or a torn frenulum linguae (remembering the possibility of non-accidental injury). The pupils are examined for their size and reflexes, remembering that a *dilated pupil may be the result of a direct injury to the eye*. The optic fundi, cranial nerves, tendon jerks and plantar reflexes are necessary parts of the neurological examination. Examination of the ear may reveal bleeding behind an intact drum. If there is bruising near the eye, the possibility of injury to the facial bones should be considered (see p. 73).

Remember the possibility of an injury to the cervical spine.

Special investigations

Clinical examination is much more important in determining what is to be done with the child than immediate X-rays taken without careful thought.

X-ray is requested *only after a full examination*. An X-ray should always be taken when a child has fallen on a sharp object, such as a broken plastic toy or a ball-point pen, when there is any penetrating injury, or when there is a possibility of a retained foreign body.

When an X-ray of the skull is thought to be necessary, the routine views are a postero-anterior, a lateral, and if there is a possibility of an occipital injury, a Towne view. If you suspect a depressed fracture ask for a tangential view and show the radiographer the area about which you are concerned. These basic views of the skull do not show the facial bones satisfactorily (see p. 74).

If non-accidental injury is suspected, a skeletal survey may be necessary (see p. 20). After a road-traffic accident, the possibility of other injuries should always be remembered, *even when there are no complaints of discomfort by a conscious child*. This applies particularly to injuries to the hips and pelvis.

Interpretation

The interpretation of the findings has been partly discussed above. Inequality of the pupils may be the result of a direct injury to the eye. A dilated pupil reacting poorly to light may suggest compression of the third nerve by oedema or haemorrhage. There may be associated weakness of the limb on the same or the opposite side or both, or decerebrate rigidity. One pupil may dilate in a fit, returning to normal when an anticonvulsant is given.

Immediately after a minor head injury a period of lethargy and drowsiness, with or without vomiting, may suggest a subdural effusion. A rise in blood pressure with slowing of the pulse and irregular breathing suggests a rise of intracranial pressure. A rapid pulse with a low blood pressure and irregular respirations may result from an occipital haemorrhage, but may be due to bleeding elsewhere or a ruptured viscus.

Bruising around the face and neck in a young child should suggest the possibility of a non-accidental injury (see p. 19).

Treatment

If the child is unconscious, the first essential is to ensure an airway. A nasogastric tube should be passed to empty the stomach. The child is then placed in the semi-prone position. *No drugs which may depress the respiratory centre or the CNS should be prescribed.*

A convulsion should be treated immediately (p. 41). For acute cerebral oedema use dexamethasone intravenously or intramuscularly, or 20% mannitol *intravenously and given very slowly* over 30–45 minutes. The dosage for dexamethasone is 2 mg for a child under three, 4 mg for a child of three to six and 8 mg for a child of six to twelve. The dosage for 20% mannitol is 50 ml for a child under three, 75 ml for a child of three to six and 100–150 ml for a child of six to twelve. The neuro-surgeon should be contacted immediately.

Children who have had a head injury should be admitted :
1   If they are known to have been unconscious.
2   If they have a fractured skull or a penetrating injury.
3   When their readings on the observation charts are going down, i.e. their level of consciousness is deteriorating.
4   If there are focal neurological signs.
5   If there is persistent vomiting.

After a minor head injury, if there is no vomiting, headache or abnormal physical signs, and there has been no loss of consciousness, a child may be allowed to go home; but no child is allowed to go home until his clinical condition is stable, after observation at intervals (recorded in the notes) for at least two hours. The parents must be told what to look for in the child's behaviour, and what symptoms or signs demand an immediate return to hospital: they include inability to awaken him, repeated vomiting, alteration of consciousness, increasing headache, unexplained crying or irritability, weakness of a limb or the development of a squint. If the child is allowed to go home, he must be seen by the doctor next day.

The decision about what is done with a child with a head injury depends much more on clinical examinations than on X-rays.

Haematoma of the scalp

A simple bruise over the skull is usually subcutaneous, and limited in extent by the firm attachment between the skin and aponeurosis.

A subaponeurotic haematoma is often extensive, covering a wide area.

A cephalhaematoma, similar to that seen in the newborn, is rare: the bleeding is between the periosteum and the bone, and is therefore confined by the attachment of the periosteum to the bone at the sutures.

Babies with a swelling on the scalp

Babies after the newborn period are not uncommonly brought with a swelling on the scalp which feels fluctuant and the edges of which feel as if there is a depression under the swelling. The story is usually that the baby is well and the mother 'just noticed the swelling' when she was brushing or washing the child's hair. There is no heat and no evidence of infection. *These babies must be X-rayed.* I have never yet seen one which did not have a skull fracture underneath. *Remember to examine the whole child because although the swelling may have resulted from a genuine accident, the possibility of non-accidental injury must always be considered* (see also p. 16). *Arrangements must always be made for the medical social worker or health visitor to follow up these children.*

Injuries of the facial bones

(See also the sections on road-traffic accidents, head injury and the teeth, pp. 67, 68 and 77.)

The precise diagnosis is often a matter for an expert but certain symptoms and signs should lead you to suspect injury and ask for help from the maxillo-facial injury unit.

Ensure an airway. A severe middle-third facial fracture may be pushed back and impacted, occluding the airway. Disimpact by inserting fingers behind the hard palate and pulling forward.

In any child with bruising round the eye it is important to determine whether a blow-out fracture of the orbit or an injury to the maxilla has occurred. The history must include the question of double vision and the direction of gaze in which this occurs. The contour of the face should be observed both from the front and also from above the child. It may be possible to palpate some alteration of contour. Any difference in the relative heights of the eyes or the pupils, any enophthalmos, ptosis or lacrimation, or disturbance of dental occlusion should be recorded. The area of a subconjunctival haemorrhage should be charted on the notes: it is particularly significant if it is not possible to see the posterior border or if the haemorrhage appears later (especially on the nasal side). If there is loss of sensation in the area supplied by the infraorbital or superior dental nerves the presence of a fracture must be assumed even although it does not show on X-ray.

The X-rays required are an occipito-mental with a 10 and 30 degree tilt, a lateral, and a lateral to show the soft tissues. Interpretation of the X-rays is difficult: look for irregularities or fracture lines near the infraorbital foramen, the zygomatic arch and the lateral wall of the antrum. Compare the line of the orbital floor with the normal side. Blood in the antrum may make it opaque.

No child with bruising around the eye should be discharged until it is clear that there is no possibility of a fracture. If there is the slightest doubt he should be seen by an ophthalmic surgeon.

Injury to the *mandible* may present with local swelling, pain, alteration in dental occlusion and difficulty in opening the mouth. Injury to the centre of the mandible may allow the tongue to fall back into the throat and obstruct the airway. Careful palpation should include palpation with the finger in the external auditory meatus when it may be possible to feel a difference in the range of movements on the two sides.

The X-rays required are a posterior–anterior view of the mandible and lateral oblique views.

Injuries to the nose which result in deformity should be seen by the ear, nose and throat surgeon. Reduction of a fracture of the nasal bones is usually done when the swelling has diminished, but the surgeon should decide the appropriate time for this.

Do not forget to tilt the child's head back to examine the nasal septum. A haematoma of the nasal septum is an emergency in a child. Treatment is urgent because if untreated it may cause necrosis of the septum. A child with a septal haematoma *must* be admitted.

Treatment of injuries of the facial bones is a matter for the experts in maxillo-facial surgery. Your responsibility is to *ensure an airway in all cases*, make careful clinical observations, record them, and know when to ask for expert help. Shock is rare in facial injuries alone and usually signifies another serious injury, e.g. a ruptured spleen.

Thoracic injuries

(See also the section on road traffic accidents, p. 67).

As in the case of all serious injuries, the detailed history is followed by assessment of the patient's condition, and full examination. An airway is ensured, a nasogastric tube passed, and if necessary, blood is taken for cross-matching. Tension pneumothorax may have to be treated as a matter of urgency. The chest is X-rayed in the supine and if possible in the upright position. If this is not possible a lateral decubitus view may have to be done. If fracture of the ribs is suspected, the site and side of the injury is noted, as this helps the radiologist to select the views to be taken. Oblique views, not lateral, are used to show rib fractures. A lung injury is more important than a rib fracture, so that the AP view of the chest is the first priority.

Pneumothorax

If there is severe dyspnoea, a needle is inserted into the second interspace anteriorly. For a tension pneumothorax in an emergency, a temporary one-way valve can be made by tying the finger of a rubber glove, with a small hole in the tip, to the

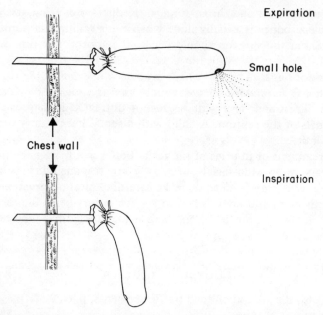

Expiration

Small hole

Chest wall

Inspiration

Fig. 9 Emergency 'one-way' value for pneumothorax made by tying the finger of a rubber glove with a small hole in the end over a large bore needle.

widest available needle until the proper equipment is available (Fig. 9).

For a haemothorax the needle is inserted into the fifth interspace in the mid-axillary line.

Abdominal injury

(See also the section road-traffic accidents, p. 67.)

Important physical signs of serious abdominal injury are shock, pain, abdominal distension, abdominal rigidity and ileus. Pain from a ruptured spleen may be referred to the left shoulder.

Awareness of the possibility of abdominal injury must be part of the examination of any injured child and the time of serial examinations and the findings must be recorded. If you find that a child with a head injury is shocked you must look for some other cause, e.g. a ruptured viscus. Supine and, if possible, erect X-ray views of the abdomen should be taken. If the child's condition makes an erect view impossible, ask for a lateral decubitus. If the child is poorly, take blood for cross-matching, set up an intravenous drip and pass a nasogastric tube before admitting him. Measure the abdominal girth at regular intervals. Further investigations are done by the surgical team.

The teeth

Broken or displaced tooth

If a tooth of the second dentition is knocked out, it can often be salvaged by reimplantation, provided that this is done promptly, within two hours of the injury, and the tooth is kept moist by immersion in normal saline. Prompt referral to the dentist (or preferably the dental hospital if there is one near) is essential. If this is impossible smear a little lignocaine anaesthetic paste on each side of the socket and after one minute inject local anaesthetic (if possible with a dental syringe and short fine needle) around the socket. Suck out the blood clot and clean it with normal saline. *Press the tooth slowly into place and hold it there for not less than ten minutes.* If no other means is available, heavy foil (e.g. a milk bottle top) can be used to mould round the area. If possible, this should be held in place by dental cement. Make arrangements for the child to be seen by a dentist, within 24 hours if possible. Remember to give tetanus toxoid if necessary. Pulp survival is good if the tooth can be reinplanted within 30 minutes. If a tooth is broken or loose, the child should be seen by the dentist the following day; but if the pulp is exposed a dental surgeon should see the child without delay, not only because of the pain but because materials are now available to protect the exposed pulp tissue and thus offer the best hope of retaining its vitality.

If after a mouth injury a tooth is lost it may be concealed in the soft tissues of the mouth or it may have been inhaled or ingested. Appropriate X-rays should be taken.

Bleeding tooth socket

The clot is removed and a small gauze pack, cut to the size of the socket, is clenched between the teeth, to apply pressure on the bleeding socket *for not less than ten minutes*. Only if necessary after that is a suture inserted under local anaesthetic (as in displaced teeth). The possibility of a blood disease should be considered if bleeding persists.

Dental abscess

This causes much pain. There may be redness and swelling over the gum, and pain on tapping the tooth, unless the nerve is dead. The child must be seen by the dentist.

Submandibular abscess

The cause must be sought; there may be an underlying tooth infection. The abscess should be drained by an incision in the line of the skin crease. If a sinus persists after drainage, an underlying dental cause should be considered.

When a child has a red painful swelling over a bone anywhere, the possibility of osteitis should be remembered.

The eyes

(See also the sections on foreign bodies and injuries to the facial bones and head, pp. 48, 73 and 68.)

Eye injuries make up only a small part of the work of paediatric Casualty, because there are no industrial injuries.

They may occur as part of a more extensive head injury or as a purely local injury, e.g. by a scratch from a thorn.

In any injury involving the eye there *must* be a precise history. The type of injuries which occur in adults when there is a penetrating injury by a piece of metal are rare, but there are many cases in which an X-ray must be done to rule out the presence of a radio-opaque foreign body which might have penetrated the orbit.

Remember to make sure that tetanus immunization is up to date.

Any eye injury in which there is loss of vision, blood in the anterior chamber (hyphema), or a laceration involving the globe, must be seen immediately by an ophthalmologist, and not just referred to the next out-patient clinic.

Eyelid injuries

You must consult the ophthalmic or plastic surgeon if an injury involves the angle between the upper and lower lids or the entrance to the nasolacrymal duct.

Chemical injury

The initial treatment of chemical injuries of the eye must be thorough irrigation with water for *at least five minutes,* if necessary holding the child face upward under a running tap. *This is extremely urgent and should take precedence over everything else.* Only after this has been done should attempts be made to get the help from the ophthalmologist, which is always necessary. A sedative may be required because the pain from a chemical injury may be considerable.

Exploding golf-ball injury

When the outer layers of a golf ball are stripped off, the semi-liquid material inside under considerable pressure may explode and cause severe injury. The eye should be X-rayed because this material is radio-opaque, and surprising quantities may be found in the periocular tissues.

Conjunctivitis

A foreign body must be looked for in any unilateral redness of the eye of recent onset (see also the section on foreign bodies, p. 48).

Bilateral 'red eyes' may be part of a viral infection in a child, perhaps by APC virus, and need no treatment.

Remember the redness and photophobia which may precede
the rash in measles. Take the temperature and look for
Koplik's spots—tiny, white spots, with a surrounding flare of
redness, near the upper molar teeth.

Purulent conjunctivitis

A swab should be taken and chloramphenicol eye drops or
ointment prescribed until the results are known. Remember
the risk of tetanus.

For severe conjunctivitis, one drop of the antibiotic should
be instilled every minute for 30 minutes, every five minutes
for the next 30 minutes, every 30 minutes for the next hour
and then a drop every two hours.

As eye drops and ointments frequently become infected,
individual containers for eye drops should be used for each
child. Any unused antibiotic eye drops should be discarded
after 14 days.

When any treatment is given for conjunctivitis the child
must be seen next day.

*Remember that sensitivity to eye drops may develop and con-
fuse the diagnosis.*

If a child with conjunctivitis complains of pain he must be
seen by an ophthalmologist, for there may be an iridocyclitis.
The same applies to the eye in which there is a leash of vessels
around the pupil.

Conjunctivitis may be due to a virus infection, such as
herpes. *Because of this, corticosteroid drops are absolutely
contraindicated for use in Casualty*. The use of corticosteroid
eye drops for a herpetic dendritic ulcer may result in loss of
the eye. *No corneal ulcer should be treated in Casualty*.

Oedema of the conjunctiva

Severe oedema of the conjunctiva is seen frequently in
children in the *hay fever* season. The swelling may be so gross
that the oedematous conjunctiva hangs out over the lower eyelids and the parents are terrified by the appearance of the eye.
In hay fever there is often intense itching of the eye, leading to

rubbing of the eye and oedema. Treatment is by instillation of 1% adrenaline eye drops (Eppy or Simplene). With the child lying down, one drop should be put into each eye and if necessary, repeated after five minutes. These cure the oedema in minutes. The possible dangers of absorption in a young child should be remembered and they should be used with great care.

An alternative treatment is by Otrivine-Antistin eye drops, instilled in the same regime as for antibiotics in severe conjunctivitis. (See the section on conjunctivitis above.)

Oedema of the conjunctiva may result from injury or allergy to eyedrops. A child may rub the eye in which there is a foreign body.

Stye

This is a self-limiting infection which does not require treatment.

Infected Meibomian cyst

This can produce enormous swelling of the affected eyelid. If it is impossible to get immediate ophthalmic help it may be necessary to relieve discomfort by incising the infected cyst after instilling 1% amethocaine. Further treatment should be given by the eye department.

Oedema of the eyelid

This may be due to a local condition such as a stye or an infected Meidomian cyst, but rarely an orbital tumour may give swelling. It may be due to inflammation in the surrounding area, e.g. an acute antrum infection, a sting, orbital cellulitis or dental abscess. *Remember that in babies swelling round the eye may indicate osteomyelitis.*

Other causes are angioneurotic oedema and allergy to eye drops or to cosmetics.

It may be caused by *drugs* of which the commonest is aspirin. Others include amitriptyline, cephaloridine, chlordiazepoxide, demeclocycline, ethosuccimide, indomethacin, nitrofurantoin, penicillin, primidone or troxidone.

Oedema of the eyelids may be the presenting symptom in dermatomyositis, infectious mononucleosis, acute nephritis and the nephrotic syndrome.

If a child presents with bilateral oedema of the eyelids remember to ask about drugs—especially aspirin. Look for rashes (purpura and urticaria) and joint swellings, examine the urine and record the blood pressure.

If the swelling is thought to be drug-induced, discontinue the drug. *Remember that antihistamines may themselves produce allergic reactions,* in some cases due to the tartrazine which is included in them.

Lacrymation

This may be due to injury, a foreign body, conjunctivitis (especially tuberculous phlyctenular conjunctivitis), hay fever, an eyelash in the canaliculum, or drugs (arsenic, mercury, nitrazepam, heroin).

Photophobia

This may be due to measles, phlyctenular conjunctivitis, ethosuccimide, troxidone or PAS.

Diplopia

Diplopia may be due to a nerve palsy (see also the section on injuries of the facial bones, p. 73). It may be caused by many drugs including antihistamines, phenytoin, nalidixic acid or primidone.

Unilateral diplopia can result from mucus associated with a meibomian cyst and also from a corneal lesion or a dislocated lens.

Blurring of vision (amblyopia)

A recent onset of blurred vision must be investigated carefully. Infection, e.g. iridocyclitis, or a foreign body should be eliminated. The onset of migraine frequently gives blurred vision.

If the optic disc and eye appear normal, blurring may result from numerous drugs, e.g. antidepressants and tranquillizers, antihistamines, chloroquine, haloperidol, isoniazid, antibiotics and antiepileptic drugs. Remember solvent-sniffing as a possible cause.

Mydriatic

For dilating the eye to examine the optic fundus, tropicamide is recommended. It has fewer side-effects than cyclopentolate. It is now available in single dose packs ('Minims').

Limb injuries
General principles

As with other conditions traumatic or otherwise, *you must take a proper history* : precisely *how* the injury occurred; the *time* it happened; whether the child was well before the accident; what previous illnesses or injuries he has had and what drugs he has been taking recently. In the case of a leg or foot injury you must ask if he walked on it after the accident or if it was immediately impossible for him to bear weight. In a young child, the precise story of the incident after which he was unable to use an arm may lead you to the correct diagnosis of a 'pulled elbow' rather than a fracture (see also p. 93). *Remember the possibility of non-accidental injury in a young child* (see also p. 16) and be sure that the history you obtain fits the clinical findings. Any young child with a limb injury should be undressed completely and examined fully.

In examining babies and young children for limb injuries you must look carefully, noticing whether he bears full weight on each leg, or limps, and whether he is using both upper limbs normally. Look for any swelling or deformity. Bruising or discoloration of the skin are usually late signs. The use of the arms is tested by using a toy or a torch to determine the range of movements. A few hours after the injury *gentle* palpation may show an area of slight warmth in a limb; this is a most useful indicator to the site of a fracture in a baby and young toddler. Feel *gently* and compare the range of movements with the normal side.

When there is an obvious deformity or swelling do not attempt to move the limb to 'see if it hurts'. Get it X-rayed first.

Remember to test the neighbouring joints for range of movement and remember that *there may be more than one fracture*, e.g. a fractured pelvis with a fractured tibia and fibula. If there is a possibility of an unstable fracture, splint the limb *before* the X-ray is taken.

Give the radiologist sufficient information, naming areas of swelling or points of maximum tenderness or heat.

The X-ray should include the whole length of the bone and the joints at both ends, otherwise fractures may be missed. This is particularly important with regard to elbow, shoulder and hip joints.

The normal variations of the epiphyseal centres frequently cause confusion: an X-ray of the opposite limb can help when interpretation is difficult but should not be done as a routine.

If it is thought that clinically there is a fracture it should be treated as such whether the X-ray shows it or not. Fractures of the scaphoid are uncommon in children but, as in adults, clinical suspicion of injury to the scaphoid should be treated as a fracture. An undisplaced fracture in, for example, an elbow may be difficult to see on the original X-rays. Remember in any elbow injury to check and recheck the radial pulse and sensation in the hand. *A child who has had an elbow injury without a fracture should not be discharged until there is full restoration of function.*

A fracture of the medial epicondyle of the humerus may be displaced into the joint and a dislocated elbow may have an associated fracture. A child with a supracondylar fracture *must be admitted* if there is any displacement.

Any child with a severely swollen elbow must be seen by the orthopaedic specialist.

Remember that a fracture confined to the shaft of the ulna is rare. There is nearly always an associated displacement of the radial head (Monteggia fracture). This is one of the occasions when it is particularly important to include the whole length of the bone.

A grossly swollen knee after a fall should be regarded as a fracture of the tibial condyle until proved otherwise, and the child must be admitted. Any fracture in a child which involves the epiphyseal plate is especially important because it may affect subsequent growth.

Even when there is a history of trauma remember the possibility of osteomyelitis or a septic arthritis. Osteomyelitis may in the early stages be clinically indistinguishable from trauma and X-rays then will usually be unhelpful.

From the medico-legal angle the most important thing is to take a full history, to examine thoroughly and to record your findings—negative as well as positive, e.g. that the child has no swelling, has a full range of movement, is bearing full weight, etc. Many unnecessary X-rays and much irradiation can be avoided.

It is most important that in any injury which has involved glass an X-ray should be taken. This does not necessarily mean that a radiographer has to be called in during the evening in all cases. Some of the children could be brought back the following morning for X-ray.

X-ray requirements

The following are suggested X-ray data for fractures (left and right should be written in full):

Hands—the digits should not be described by number, but by name, e.g. thumb, index finger, ring finger, etc. This is a Medical Defence Union recommendation, resulting from numerous claims arising from operations on a wrong digit. The standard views for both hands and feet are AP and oblique.

Wrists—the standard views are AP, lateral, and if necessary oblique.

Scaphoid—in addition to the above a special 'scaphoid' view is requested. A fracture may not be visible immediately after the injury. If a fracture is suspected clinically, it should be treated as such.

Elbows—the head of the radius should be opposite the epiphysis or the capitellum in all views. If there is any doubt about the diagnosis the opposite side should be taken for comparison.

Ankles—the standard views are AP and lateral. Oblique views may be necessary to diagnose a fracture of the medial malleolus.

Cervical spine—if an injury is suspected, an AP, lateral and an AP through-mouth view should be taken. In children an X-ray of the cervical spine taken in flexion may show apparent subluxation, which is disproved by a further X-ray taken with the neck extended (see Fig. 10 and the section on acute neck stiffness, p. 134).

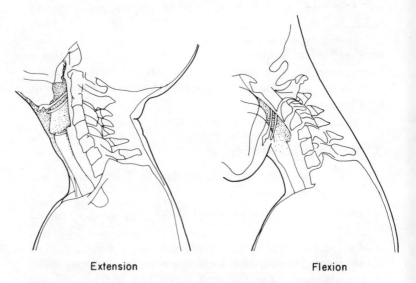

Extension   Flexion

Fig. 10 In children an X-ray of the cervical spine taken in flexion may show apparent subluxation, which is disproved by a further X-ray taken with the neck extended.

Treatment

All children with fractures, who are allowed home after treatment, *must be seen in the fracture clinic the following day.* Some of the children who have a general anaesthetic for manipulation of a fracture may be allowed home after recovery from the anaesthetic, but many will need to be admitted if the manipulation has been difficult, if there has to be a considerable delay because the child has eaten recently or if it is late in the evening. Regional blocks are not used in small children.

Summary of recommended treatment

	Treatment	Comments
Upper limb injuries		
Clavicle and shoulder		
Sterno-clavicular dislocation	Sling	
Acromio-clavicular dislocation	Sling	
Soft-tissue injuries of shoulder	Sling	
Dislocation of shoulder	Manipulate under anaesthetic (MUA) Collar and cuff sling inside clothes	Possible nerve injury, especially with posterior dislocation
Clavicle fracture	Figure of eight bandage: adjust frequently	May need sling as well for few days at first
Scapular fractures	Sling	
Humerus :		
Surgical neck		
Undisplaced	Inside collar and cuff	
Displaced	Senior orthopaedic help	Easily missed, may trap deltoid
Shaft fractures		
Undisplaced	Collar and cuff with gutter splint or U-slab under clothes	Get orthopaedic help for any which are displaced or with neurovascular damage
Displaced	Senior orthopaedic help	

	Treatment	Comments

Elbow—Any very swollen elbow must be seen by the orthopaedic department :

Supracondylar fracture

	Treatment	Comments
Undisplaced	Inside collar and cuff	
Displaced	Refer for senior orthopaedic help for M U A and admission	**Check radial pulse repeatedly.** *These must be admitted.*

Lateral condyle

Undisplaced	Inside collar and cuff	
Displaced	Admit. May need open reduction	Admit at once

Medial epicondyle

Undisplaced	Inside collar and cuff	
Displaced	Admit for M U A or open reduction	May give ulnar nerve symptoms. X-ray opposite elbow for comparison if necessary

Dislocated elbow

Uncomplicated	M U A **as soon as possible.** Inside collar and cuff	Admit after reduction
Fracture dislocation	**Admit.** Needs senior orthopaedic help	

Ulna :
Olecranon fracture

Undisplaced	Full arm plaster of Paris (P O P) and sling	
Displaced	Admit	

Ulnar shaft

Undisplaced	Full arm P O P and sling	*Must have complete views of radius and ulna including elbow and wrist joints*
Monteggia (fractured ulnar shaft and displacement of head)	Senior help for M U A and full arm P O P	Isolated ulnar shaft fracture is very rare

Ulnar head

Undisplaced	Dorsal P O P slab and sling	
Displaced	M U A, full arm P O P and sling	
Ulnar styloid	Dorsal forearm P O P slab	

Treatment	Comments	
Radius:		
Head and neck		
Undisplaced crack	Inside collar and cuff	
Head		
Displaced or comminuted	Senior help for reduction under anaesthetic. Inside collar and cuff	
Shaft (isolated fracture)		
Undisplaced	Full arm P O P and sling	
Displaced	M U A, full arm P O P and sling	
Distal radius		
Simple greenstick fractures of the radius alone	Full arm P O P with forearm in full supination or full pronation	They have a bad reputation and *often deform later*. Position must be checked by X-ray weekly until healed
Displaced	As above after M U A	
Fracture dislocations and epiphyseal separations	Needs senior orthopaedic help	
Radius and ulna:		
Midshaft fracture		
Undisplaced	Full arm P O P	
Displaced	Will need senior orthopaedic help for reduction under anaesthetic	
Distal radius and ulna		
Undisplaced greenstick	Dorsal slab and sling	
Displaced greenstick	*Gentle* M U A . Full arm P O P	
Completely displaced	Get senior help	

All wringer and spin-dryer injuries + or − fractures must be admitted for 24 hours

Carpus:		
Scaphoid	Scaphoid plaster	Treat on *clinical* findings even if X-ray negative

	Treatment	**Comments**
Other undisplaced carpal fractures	Scaphoid P O P	

All *displacements* or fracture dislocations need senior orthopaedic help

Metacarpals :

First metacarpal

	Treatment	**Comments**
Undisplaced	Scaphoid type plaster	
Displaced, into joint, or dislocation of carpo-metacarpal joint	M U A. Scaphoid type plaster	

Other metacarpals

Undisplaced	Dorsal P O P slab or mitten bandage with fingers slightly flexed over pad	
Displaced	M U A	If very displaced may need internal fixation

Metacarpophalangeal joint dislocations (except first)	Strap to next finger	
First metacarpophalangeal joint dislocation	M U A and extended scaphoid type plaster	Check radial and ulnar collateral ligaments— may need open reduction if tendons are trapped

Proximal and intermediate phalanges

Undisplaced	Strap to next finger	
Displaced	M U A. Zimmer splint or plaster shell used with care with fingers slightly flexed	Make sure that there is no rotation by flexing the fingers and looking at the position of the fingernails
Thumb fractures	Extended scaphoid type P O P	

Lower limb injuries

Femur	All femoral fractures need admission. Apply Thomas splint *before* X-ray	Sedate before X-ray

Patella

Undisplaced fracture	Robert Jones bandage or padded P O P cylinder —*only* after senior advice	No weight bearing

	Treatment	Comments
Displaced	Admit	
Dislocation patella	M U A. Robert Jones bandage or P O P cylinder after senior advice	No weight bearing
Knee	Any haemarthrosis or dislocation *must be admitted*	
Tibia :		
Spine and condyles	Admit	
Shaft		
Undisplaced	Full leg P O P *with knee flexed 15°*	
Displaced	M U A and full leg P O P as above	Admit
Distal epiphyseal fracture		
Displaced	Needs senior orthopaedic help	
Fibula :		
Shaft in isolation	Below knee P O P	X-ray ankle
Shaft with diastasis	M U A by senior orthopaedic help—full leg P O P	
Ankle injuries :		
No fracture and full weight bearing	Strapping	**Take proper history** re weight-bearing, circumstances of accident. **Examine os calcis.** If in doubt review in one or two days
No fracture but severe discomfort	Below knee walking P O P	If discomfort continues remember possibility of osteomyelitis. If there are *signs on both sides of the ankle, check stability before applying plaster*
Avulsion fractures of either malleolar tips	Below knee walking P O P	

	Treatment	Comments
Fracture of either malleolus		
Undisplaced	Below knee *resting* P O P	
Displaced	Get senior orthopaedic help	
Bi or tri-malleolar fractures	Admit	
Os calcis	Wool and crepe bandage No weight bearing Admit if bilateral	*Examine hips, spine and neck*
Talus		
Undisplaced	Below knee resting P O P	
Displaced or dislocated	Admit	
Chip fractures of *navicular* or neck of talus	Below knee walking P O P	
Metatarsals		
First	Below knee resting P O P	
Others	Below knee walking P O P	
Phalanges	Metatarsal bar and padded bandage on toe	

X-ray hips and pelvis in femoral fractures and in serious lower leg injuries

Further reading

POLLEN A. *Fractures and Dislocations in Children.* London: Churchill Livingstone, 1973.

RANG M. *Children's Fractures.* New York: Lippincott, 1974.

SHARRARD W.J.W. *Paediatric Orthopaedics and Fractures.* 2nd edn. Oxford: Blackwell Scientific Publications, 1979.

Wringer and spin-dryer injuries to the arms

These must always be taken seriously and every case should be admitted for at least 24 hours so that the arm can be elevated and observed.

Fractures often occur with spin-dryers but in wringer injuries fractures are uncommon. In a series of 557 cases (Stone *et al.* 1976) there were no fractures. The injuries consist of friction burns, contusions, bruises, lacerations and dislocation of the metacarpophalangeal joint. If the injury reaches up to the axilla there may be nerve injuries. Skin grafting of the area of the friction burns may be needed later.

The most dangerous feature is the tremendous swelling which can occur some hours after the injury and which can lead to severe tissue damage and even gangrene, if it is not anticipated by admission for elevation of the arm and careful monitoring.

Further reading

STONE H.H., CANTWELL D.V. & FUTENWIDER J.T. Wringer arm injuries. *J. Pediatr. Surg.* 1976, **11**:375.

Pulled elbow

It is common to see a young child who has been brought because he 'has suddenly lost the use of one arm' and has obvious discomfort.

The diagnosis of a 'pulled elbow' can nearly always be made by taking a precise and careful history and can be confirmed by the physical examination.

The head of the radius is pulled partially through the annular ligament; the child loses the use of his arm and has pain. It may result from the parents swinging the child by his arms in play, dragging the refractory toddler against his will or pulling him up off the ground by the outstretched arms. It can occasionally happen when the child falls but continues to hold on to a static object which acts as the pulling force. Two of the alternative names for this condition, 'temper-tantrum elbow' or 'nurse maid's elbow' emphasize the cause. It occurs predominantly in the one- to three-year-old age group, but can be found up to the age of six. The condition is often a recurrent one.

In a study of 100 cases, it was found that the site of the pain, in children who were old enough to locate it, was in the elbow in 53, in the elbow and shoulder in 6, in the elbow and forearm in 3, in the shoulder alone in 3, in the forearm alone in 11 and in the wrist in 23. This example of referred pain is a common source of diagnostic error. On examination there is no swelling of the elbow, and no loss of elbow flexion, but slight limitation of full supination of the forearm. The X-ray is normal.

The condition is treated by simple manipulation without anaesthetic, the doctor holding the lower part of the humerus firmly, and with the thumb over the head of the radius, rapidly flicking the forearm into full supination. Nearly always there is a palpable click. Re-examine the child in five to ten minutes, when it is usual to find that he has forgotten all about the injury. No sling or other treatment is required. Occasionally more than one manipulation may be needed.

Further reading

ILLINGWORTH C.M. Pulled elbow—a study of 100 patients. *Br. med. J.* 1975; ii:672.

Trapped fingers and amputated fingertips

These are common injuries in a paediatric casualty department. They vary in degree from slight swelling of the fingertip to a guillotine amputation of the tip. In my experience, no injury causes more distress to the parents, who in addition may feel guilty because they have themselves trapped the fingers in a car door.

If they are dealt with as outlined below, excellent results can be obtained with minimum discomfort to the children.

Trapped fingertips with partial avulsion

(see Figs 11 and 12)

It is *never* necessary to suture trapped fingers; in any case, crushed tissue takes sutures very badly.

1 They should be cleaned gently, repositioned and held in place by Steristrip or Ethistrip which is applied beginning from the surface of the finger where the tip is still partially attached. A space *must* be left between the strips. The ends of

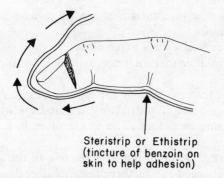

Steristrip or Ethistrip
(tincture of benzoin on
skin to help adhesion)

Fig. 11 Method of repositioning a trapped finger with partial avulsion. Application of Steristrip or Ethistrip on the surface of the finger where the tip is still partially attached.

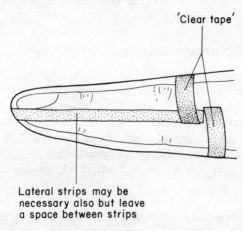

'Clear tape'

Lateral strips may be
necessary also but leave
a space between strips

Fig. 12 The ends of the strips are anchored by 'Clear tape'.

the strips are anchored by 'Clear tape'. (See also the section on lacerations, p. 45.) In most cases this should be done by the doctor, but in any case *the position must be checked by the doctor*.

2   In all cases leave the nail in position.

3   **Do not put strips all round the finger.** They will not stretch if the finger swells.

4   Put on a *non-adherent* dressing (Melolin or similar).

5   Over this put on a mitten bandage.

6   Check that the immunizations are up-to-date and *do not give any antibiotics*.

7   Leave for *at least* a week to ten days.

8   Warn the mother that the finger will look awful at the first dressing.

9   In seven to ten days remove the top dressings only, leaving the strips in position if satisfactory and redress with a *non-adherent* dressing as before. The finger often looks slimy at this stage.

10   After another seven to ten days remove all the strips, etc. Very few fingers need any further dressings after this.

11   Do not discharge until you are satisfied that function is full.

12   Warn the mother that the fingertip will look redder than the others for several weeks.

Guillotine amputations of fingertips

Terminal amputations of fingertips in young children do extremely well with conservative treatment only. Even if the bone protrudes slightly it should be left alone.

1   The finger should be cleaned gently.

2   The finger is covered with *several layers* of Tulle Gras or Jelonet and a mitten bandage is applied.

3   Do not give any antibiotics but check tetanus immunization.

4   Leave alone for *at least a fortnight*.

5   Warn the mother that it will look awful at the first dressing but should do very well.

6   In a fortnight repeat the same dressing and review in another two weeks. Usually three to four dressings are required. There should be regrowth of the tip and nail and complete restoration of function with an excellent cosmetic result eventually, provided that the amputation is distal to the distal interphalangeal joint (Fig. 13).

Subungual haematoma

If this is painful, relief is given by releasing the blood by trephining the nail—by heating the end of a metal paper clip

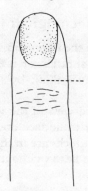

Fig. 13 Guillotine amputation of the finger-tip. An amputated tip distal to the dotted line should regenerate well in children.

and holding it against the nail or by using a tiny electric drill made for the purpose.

A subungual haematoma which is not painful should be left alone.

When a fingernail is beginning to separate it may look as if a paronychia is developing and this can be a trap for the unwary. It seems to be caused by the skin being stretched over the most proximal part of the separating nail, giving a creamy-yellow appearance which may resemble pus.

Further reading

ILLINGWORTH C.M. Trapped fingers and amputated fingertips in children. *J. Pediatr. Surg.* 1974; **9**:853.

Mitten injuries

Mann (1961) described necrosis of the fingertip as a result of a nylon (or woollen) thread from a mitten becoming entwined round the finger and causing constriction of the fingertip; gangrene may result.

Further reading

MANN T. Fingertip necrosis in the newly born. A hazard of wearing mittens. *Br. med. J.* 1961; **ii**:1755.

Gynaecological injury

Trauma which involves the perineum in a child, except for the most trivial superficial abrasion or bruising, will usually need examination under an anaesthetic by a gynaecologist or a paediatric surgeon.

In a young girl a good view of the vagina and cervix can be obtained by getting her to lie face downwards with the knees pulled up so that the buttocks are in the air. If the buttocks are held apart an auroscope head (without a speculum) will give a good view.

Criminal injury

(See also the section on if you have to go to court, p. 25.)

The doctor should seek the help of the forensic pathologist. The clothing should be placed in a labelled, sealed bag for examination for blood, sperm and hair; if this is handed to the police, ask for a signed receipt.

The child is examined for bruises, scratches and other trauma. *The notes must be carefully made at the time of the examination, and should include sketches of any findings, and if possible, photographs.*

For vaginal examination under an anaesthetic, the help of the gynaecologist or paediatric surgeon should be sought.

It is important that the doctor should tell the parents about the importance of not talking about the incident to the child after she returns home. Much of the psychological trauma of sexual attacks can be traced to parental anxiety and constant expressions of that anxiety to the child.

Stings and bites

(See also the section on anaphylaxis, p. 66.)

Stings

There is no specific treatment (alkali, acid or anything else) for a wasp or bee sting. Application of gauze pads dipped in iced water may give some relief. For a severe allergic reaction one would give 1 in 1000 adrenaline by intramuscular injection (and chlorpheniramine by mouth) and a bronchodilator if there are asthmatic symptoms, but normally no treatment is required.

The treatment for a jellyfish sting is similar.

If a child has severe allergic reactions to stings, the parents should be provided with adrenaline for injection in an emergency. A suitable outfit, which includes a syringe, is made by IMS (the Min-I-Jet System).

Dog bites

Dog or cat bites are treated like any other penetrating wound. Remember tetanus prophylaxis.

Rabies

This has spread greatly in recent years to Germany, Holland, Switzerland, Belgium and France. The animals infected are not just dogs and cats but include foxes and other animals.

Human diploid vaccine is now obtainable and this can be used both for prophylactic immunization and for treatment following suspected rabies contact.

If someone has been bitten when abroad or bitten by a biting animal smuggled into this country, action is urgent. The incubation period can vary from as little as ten days in a bite on the head and neck to as long as a year after a bite on a foot.

Record:

1   The date of the bite.
2   The part of the body bitten or scratched with a description of the injury.
3   The exact address at which it happened.
4   Details of the dog and name and address of the dog owner if known.
5   Whether the incident was reported to the local doctor or police.
6   Details of any treatment given abroad.

Contact the nearest public health laboratory for advice and a supply of vaccine. If there is difficulty the Virus Reference Laboratory (Tel. 01-205-7041) will help. The DHSS have links with Europe and may be able to give information about the rabies position in the area where the bite occurred, and the present state of the biting dog.

Recent wounds

The wound should be washed immediately and it should be flushed with soap and water. After the soap has been washed off 40–70% alcohol, tincture of iodine or 0·1% quaternary ammonium compound should be applied. Anti-rabies serum should, if possible, be instilled into the depth of the wound and infiltrated around it. Suturing should if possible be postponed.

Rabies vaccine

The first injection of anti-rabies vaccine should be given as soon as possible, 1 ml either intramuscularly or by deep subcutaneous injection.

Three further doses should be given on the third, seventh and fourteenth day and booster injections at one and three months. If the biting animal can be proved to be rabies-free ten days after the event, the injections can be stopped.

Snake bite

The adder bite is the usual snake bite in the UK. It causes much pain and anxiety but serious results are rare. **Immobilize the bitten limb.** The bitten part is cleaned, a cold compress applied, and a sedative given. Recovery is usually rapid.

When snake bites do occur there may be vomiting, abdominal pain and diarrhoea within a few minutes. The most important sign of severe adder poisoning is hypotension, but there may be ECG changes and a neutrophil leucocytosis.

If there is vomiting, the child is placed in the prone position, and prochlorperazine may be prescribed. An alternative is an antihistamine, such as promethazine, or 100 mg of hydrocortisone intramuscularly (10–25 mg at the age of six to twelve years).

The refined (Zagreb) anti-venom which is now available is much less likely to give severe anaphylactoid reactions but adrenaline 1 in 1000 solution should nevertheless be available in a syringe.

Indications for anti-venom

1 Bleeding from the gums, nose or any other site distant from the bite itself, which started spontaneously after the bite.
2 Failure of the patient's blood to clot if placed in a clear, dry glass tube and left for 30 minutes.
3 *Massive* swelling of the bitten limb (more than half the limb being involved).
4 Signs of nervous system involvement, extreme drowsiness, dysphagia and difficulty in breathing.
5 Signs of heart involvement, a low BP, an unusually slow pulse rate or irregular rhythm, and an abnormal ECG.

Give no more than 2 ampoules (10 ml) *very slowly*. It should be diluted in 50–100 ml of saline. *Do not incise the site* of the bite; doing so can give severe blood loss. The anti-venom is obtained from Guy's Hospital Poisons Centre (Tel. 01-407-7600) and designated regional centres.

Absence of swelling at the site of the bite four hours after indicates that no venom was injected and therefore no treatment is indicated.

Advice on the management of bites and stings can be obtained from the Liverpool School of Tropical Medicine, Pembroke Place, Liverpool L3 5QA (Tel. 051-708-9393).

Part 3

Introduction
Disease in immigrant children:
 illness after holidays abroad
Any acute illness
The crying baby
Pyrexia of unknown origin
Acute abdominal pain
Abdominal distension
Vomiting
Diarrhoea
Blood in the stool
Rectal prolapse
The skin
   Nappy rash
   Scabies
   Papular urticaria
   'Hand, foot and mouth' disease
   Chicken-pox
   Molluscum contagiosum
   Bullous eruptions
   Exfoliative dermatitis
   Impetigo
   Boils
   Pediculosis capitis (nits)
   Purpura
   Sunburn
   Erythema nodosum
   Other skin conditions
Other causes of pruritus
Oedema
Swelling of the face
Headache and neurological symptoms
Symptoms in the ear, nose and throat
Some respiratory symptoms
Some genitourinary symptoms
Limp and limb pains
Swelling of a joint: arthritis

Introduction

In this section I have picked out some of the common or more important symptoms of disease met with in a casualty department, giving the chief causes, the important difficulties in diagnosis, and, where relevant, the management.

Even though the final diagnosis may not be made in the casualty department or in the surgery, I think it adds to the interest of the work if the doctor examining the child has a reasonable knowledge of the possible causes. Potentially serious mistakes may be avoided if he knows the conditions which need further investigation by a paediatrician or paediatric surgeon.

For further details of common symptoms, see Illingworth (1982).

Disease in immigrant children: illness after holidays abroad

Coloured immigrant children may have diseases rarely seen in British children. It is important to know whether they were born abroad and when they were last in their country of origin. If they have lived in these countries they may harbour a variety of worms, of which ankylostoma, amongst others, is an important cause of debility. If they have been in their home country recently, malaria, enteric fever and even cholera have to be considered. Dermal Leishmaniasis is common in parts of Iraq, causing ulceration and scarring on the face or elsewhere. Tuberculosis, now generally unconsidered in British children, certainly has to be considered in coloured children not born in this country.

Sickle cell anaemia occurs amongst American negroes, in parts of India, the West Indies and large parts of Africa: it has such protean manifestations that it has certainly to be remembered in the case of coloured children. Thalassaemia occurs in the Mediterranean area, India, Pakistan and Ceylon: it causes anaemia with splenomegaly. Glucose 6 phosphate dehydrogenase deficiency occurs in Greeks, Cypriots, Turks, Chinese,

Indians, Saudi Arabians, Filipinos, and Jews from Iraq and Iran. Haemolysis may occur when the child is given anti-malarial drugs, diphenhydramine, nitrofurantoin, salicylates, sulphonamides, Vitamin K or other drugs, or when he eats broad beans or acquires certain infections.

When British children are seen because of illness following a holiday in countries abroad the possibilities to consider are the enteric, dysentery and Salmonella group, malaria and polio-myelitis. Visceral Leishmaniasis, giving PUO and hepato-megaly, can occur after a visit to Malta or other parts of the Mediterranean area from a bite by sandflies.

Any acute illness

The history

The general principles of history-taking have been discussed on p. 6.

When a child presents with an acute illness, it is essential to know its exact duration, and when the child was last perfectly well—and in particular whether he has had the symptoms before. One needs to know whether anyone else in the family (or school friend) has the same symptoms or whether there has been any contact with an infectious disease, what medicines (prescribed or unprescribed) the child has been given (including aspirin), whether there has been a recent immuni-zation, and whether he has recently been abroad. One has to ask *specifically* about every system of the body—the nose for nasal discharge, the ear for pain or discharge, the throat, the chest for a cough, the stomach for vomiting, the bowels for diarrhoea, and the urinary system for frequency, scalding, etc. One asks whether the child has pain anywhere.

If the child has a pain, one needs to have answers to the following questions:
1　Where is the pain?
2　Is it always in the same place? The pain of appendicitis may begin in the periumbilical region, and then settle in the right iliac fossa. Otherwise pain which is located first in one place and then in another is less likely to be organic.

3 How severe is it? One wants to know whether it makes the child cry, doubles him up, stops him playing, keeps him awake, or takes him off his food. One asks the mother, 'Would you know that he had the pain if he did not tell you? If the answer is no, it is not likely to be severe.

4 Is it getting better or worse?

5 What brings the pain on, what relieves it? A pleural pain is worse on inspiration.

6 What sort of pain is it? A pleural or peritoneal pain is often stabbing and knife-like in nature.

7 Is it continuous or intermittent? A rhythmical pain coming and going every few minutes suggests an intestinal origin. A child too young to describe it may have episodes in which he looks pale and poorly and then recovers.

8 If the pain comes in attacks, how frequent are the attacks, how long do they last, and are they coming more or less frequently? One often finds that the recurrent pain about which the mother is worried lasts moments only, and occurs once every three or four months: it is then not likely to be serious.

9 Are there any associated symptoms, e.g. headache, bowel or urinary symptoms?

For the routine examination and for special investigations see pp. 7–10.

The crying baby

A distinction must be made between the baby who is said to be 'constantly crying' and has done so for a long time, from the child who is crying with an acute illness.

The usual causes for 'constant crying', other than an acute illness, are hunger, excessive wind (due to too small a hole in the teat if bottle fed), thirst due to overconcentrated feeds, evening colic (first three or four months only), boredom, the desire to be picked up, excessive heat or cold, or an itchy rash. Often no cause can be found and it is assumed that the problem is one of his developing personality. An erupting tooth, untreated coeliac disease or phenylketonuria, and perhaps other metabolic defects, may also present with crying.

When a child is brought on account of constant crying, and none of the usual causes can be found, it is important to remember that the mother may be becoming worn out, and that this is a 'pre-battering' situation.

The sudden development of constant crying in a baby previously well but now ill, may be due to otitis media, urinary tract infection, meningitis or other infection, alimentary tract obstruction, subdural effusion or torsion of a testis.

Pyrexia of unknown origin

When the obvious causes of fever have been eliminated, including in particular otitis media, tonsillitis, urinary tract infection or the onset of an acute infectious disease such as measles, infectious mononucleosis, roseola infantum or enteric fever there remain many possible diagnoses to consider. The possibility of meningitis must not be forgotten.

In the newborn, an E. coli or similar septicaemia is an important condition to eliminate. Chronic dehydration, due to one of the causes of polyuria, may cause a rise of temperature. Meningococcal septicaemia may present with high fever, and later on arthritis and a few petechial haemorrhages. Tuberculosis can usually be eliminated by a tuberculin test, but not always, for the test may be negative in miliary tuberculosis and temporarily negative in measles or other infections: choroidal tubercles can be seen in two out of three children with miliary tuberculosis, and the X-ray of the chest may help to establish the diagnosis of tuberculosis, later confirmed by stomach washings and urine examination.

A perinephric or subphrenic abscess would normally be the sequel of appendicitis. Examination of all bones for tenderness or for areas of slight local warmth with blood cultures, help to eliminate osteitis. Subacute bacterial endocarditis is usually associated with congenital heart disease, of which there are usually signs. Fever may be a manifestation of chronic liver disease, leukaemia or malignant tumours. Prolonged unexplained fever may precede the obvious manifestations of rheumatoid arthritis by many months. Rarer infections to eliminate

include toxocara, in which there is often eosinophilia, and toxoplasmosis.

Fever may be a side-effect of numerous drugs. Malingering
is a rare cause of elevation of the temperature. By various
means, including rapid rubbing of the bulb of the thermometer, the unwary may be deceived. However, a normal white
cell count and normal ESR help to eliminate many of the
infections. Very occasionally a child has a slightly raised temperature, is well, and nothing abnormal is found after full
investigation.

Acute abdominal pain

General principles

No symptom presents a greater challenge to the casualty
doctor or the family doctor than acute abdominal pain in
children. Probably all children sooner or later experience some
abdominal pain. The possible causes are innumerable, and in
this section I shall discuss some of the more important ones
and some of the difficulties in diagnosis.

The importance of a full history has been discussed on p. 6.
One must know when the child had his last bowel action, and
whether he is passing flatus. Enquiry should be made about an
upper respiratory tract infection in the last few days, and, in
all cases, about medicines taken by the child—for they may be
the cause of the pain.

The examination (p. 7) must be a full one. The *whole body* is
inspected, e.g. for a rash, such as that of anaphylactoid purpura which often predominantly affects the buttocks. The
abdomen is inspected *before palpation* for distension and peristalsis. As already emphasized, when palpating the abdomen
one watches the child's face for evidence of tenderness on
palpation. One auscultates for peristaltic sounds. In all cases
the genitalia are examined for a strangulated hernia or torsion
of a testis, and in all cases a rectal examination is required.

The most useful special investigations are usually the white cell count, ESR, urine examination and culture, and where relevant, examination for sickle cell anaemia.

Abdominal pain is regarded particularly seriously if there is also vomiting, if it has lasted for over three hours, if the child looks ill or if the temperature is raised. It is more likely to be significant if the pain is localized than if it is diffuse. A fairly severe pain may precede the development of diarrhoea: and pain may result from a bad cough or from vomiting. *The presence of diarrhoea by no means excludes the diagnosis of acute appendicitis or peritonitis or intussusception.* The finding of an excess of white cells in a centrifuged specimen of urine must not be thought to prove the presence of pyelonephritis; it may occur in pelvic peritonitis and appendicitis. The ESR is often normal in anaphylactoid purpura.

No child with acute abdominal pain should be sent home by a casualty doctor without a senior doctor seeing the child. He may have to be re-examined after an interval. If it is thought that he is fit to go home, the family doctor is told on the telephone, the parents are told to bring the child back immediately if there is any reason for anxiety or deterioration, and in any case the child *must be seen next day*.

Recurrent abdominal pain

This common condition affects mainly school-age children. Many have attacks of central abdominal pain with vomiting, pallor and often fever. It may be related to migraine. The pain may be very severe. In 94% of cases no organic cause is found: but in the remaining 6% the cause may lie in hydronephrosis, recurrent volvulus, urinary tract infection, peptic ulcer or other cause. It is *not* due to a 'grumbling appendix' or 'chronic appendicitis'. The danger in making the diagnosis when a child has had several attacks is the possibility that the present attack is due to a different cause, such as acute appendicitis. It follows that however many attacks the child may have had, a full history and examination are essential. If the attack has passed at the time of examination the parents should be told to bring the child back *as soon as another attack has begun*.

Acute appendicitis

It would be much easier for the doctor if all children with acute appendicitis had the symptoms of abdominal pain, vomiting, constipation and fever, the pain commencing in the umbilical area and settling down in the right iliac fossa. Unfortunately the diagnosis is often more difficult. In several studies it was found that about 10% have dysuria (and there may be an excess of white cells and some albumin in the urine) and about 10% have diarrhoea. Appendicitis can occur at any age, and infants with acute appendicitis usually present with diarrhoea, urinary symptoms and an abdominal mass, often with acetone in the urine, and the white cell count may be normal, though this is unusual. In 40% of 100 cases of perforated appendix, there had been no localization of pain. When the appendix is retrocaecal, the pain may be in the upper part of the abdomen on the right, or not localized. Occasionally the pain may be in the left iliac fossa. In some cases there is no pain at all. The temperature is not usually high, but may be over 39° in an occasional case.

It may be difficult or impossible to distinguish acute appendicitis from acute mesenteric lymphadenitis.

Intussusception

If all children with intussusception were aged three to nine months, had had severe rhythmical attacks of abdominal pain, vomiting and pallor, with blood in the stool and a palpable sausage-shaped mass, the diagnosis would be easier. Unfortunately there are many variations from this picture: there may be a normal bowel action on the first day, or even diarrhoea; there is often no blood in the stool; in 10% or more there is no pain, but attacks of severe pallor with or without vomiting; and in 10% there is a history of a preceding upper respiratory tract infection; in 10% there may be a high white cell count; and in about 15% the temperature is raised.

When a child is said to have had one or more attacks of 'looking awful' and perhaps going limp, it is often difficult to decide whether the cause is something like intussusception or if he has had a fit.

Torsion of the testis

This occurs at any age including infancy: the pain may be abdominal or scrotal and often in the groin. *An acute painful swelling in the scrotum should be diagnosed as torsion of the testis until proved otherwise, and referred urgently to the surgeon for exploration.* Epididymoorchitis is extremely rare unless associated with a chronic urinary tract infection, and the orchitis of mumps is very rare before puberty.

Pain from the urinary tract

The causes include pyelonephritis, hydronephrosis, renal calculus and acute nephritis. The latter can cause abdominal pain.

Other causes of acute abdominal pain

These include pneumonia and pleurisy (pain being referred to the abdomen), infective hepatitis, Meckel's diverticulitis, acute rheumatic fever, sickle cell anaemia, anaphylactoid purpura, and diabetes or associated hypoglycaemia. A pancreatic pseudocyst may develop around a month after an upper abdominal injury, causing pain and vomiting.

Investigations

These must depend on the history and examination, but the most useful ones will usually be microscopy of urine and culture, and a blood count. If there is a possibility of obstruction, erect and supine views of the abdomen may show fluid levels. *Do not treat as a urinary tract infection until it has been proved to be one.*

Further reading

APLEY J. *The Child with Abdominal Pains.* Oxford: Blackwell Scientific Publications, 1975.
AULDIST A.W. Appendicitis in patients under five years of age. *Aust. Paediatr. J.* 1967; **3**:144.

EIN S.H., STEPHENS C.A. & MINOR A. The painless intussusception. *J. Pediatr. Surg.* 1976; **11**:563.

PENA S.D.J. & MEDOVY H. Child abuse and traumatic pseudocyst of the pancreas. *J. Pediatr.* 1973; **83**:1026.

RAVITCH M.M. Consideration of errors in the diagnosis of intussusception. *Am. J. Dis. Child.* 1952; **84**:17.

Abdominal distension

In the *newborn* period, a perforation in the alimentary or urinary tract should be considered, as well as tumours, cysts and hydronephrosis. Perforation of the stomach is manifested by abdominal distension, vomiting, respiratory distress and melaena, usually around the third day of life. A perforation in the urinary tract, causing ascites, is usually the result of urethral obstruction. One of the features of chloramphenicol toxicity in the newborn (the grey syndrome) is abdominal distension, associated with cyanosis and pallor. In Hirschsprung's disease there is usually abdominal distension, often with alternating constipation and diarrhoea.

When the child is older abdominal distension, more than that commonly seen in the normal toddler, may be due to steatorrhoea, gross constipation, ascites or tumour. Diphenoxylate (Lomotil) should not be used in children but can be a cause of otherwise unexplained distension.

Intestinal obstruction may present with abdominal pain (with or without vomiting) and some localized distension of the abdomen (see the section on acute abdominal pain above).

Vomiting

Because innumerable conditions cause vomiting in childhood, I have picked out some particularly important features and conditions as a guide to diagnosis.

Probably all children vomit sooner or later. *Features of particular importance* include the following:

1 Green, bile-stained vomitus. In the newborn this indicates intestinal obstruction until proved otherwise.

2 Persistent vomiting, as distinct from intermittent vomiting.

3 The child becoming unwell, suckling less well, loss of

appetite, ceasing to smile (after five or six weeks of age) and
drowsiness.
4 Abdominal distension.
5 Visible peristalsis.
6 Dehydration.
7 Loss of weight.
8 Fever.
9 Headache associated with vomiting.

Newborn

Obstruction may be caused by a meconium plug (often dealt
with simply by inserting the little finger in the rectum), oesophageal atresia (in which case there may have been hy-
dramnios, and the baby is obviously unable to swallow mucus
and saliva), duodenal atresia (in which case there is severe
vomiting but without abdominal distension) or obstruction
farther down the alimentary tract. In Hirschsprung's disease
there is often a story that no stool was passed in the first 24
hours and there is constipation or alternating severe diarrhoea
and constipation, with abdominal distension: on rectal examination the rectum is empty.

Intracranial causes include cerebral oedema or haemorrhage, subdural effusion or meningitis. Fullness of the
fontanelle and wide separation of the sutures may point to an
intracranial cause, but in meningitis *there may be no bulging of
the fontanelle or neck stiffness :* the child is just ill, and there is
no other discoverable cause. E. coli septicaemia is another
important cause of vomiting and illness in the newborn: there
may or may not be evidence of umbilical infection.

Urethral obstruction in the male is manifested by a poor
stream of urine and a palpable bladder. Other causes which
are rare but treatable are galactosaemia and adrenocortical hyperplasia. In the latter there may or may not be notable enlargement of the phallus; biochemical investigation will establish the diagnosis.

Infants after the newborn period

Almost all babies bring a small amount of milk up after a feed:

some do it more than others. A major cause of vomiting is excess of wind, which in a bottle-fed baby is almost always due to too small a hole in the teat. Congenital pyloric stenosis presents almost always between three and eight weeks of age with the story of one large vomit immediately after or during a feed. Peristalsis can often be seen, and a pea-sized tumour can almost always be felt. After ten weeks of age it is exceedingly rare. The ruminator is hardly likely to present in a casualty department: the baby arches the back and tries to bring the milk up and he may appear to gargle with the milk in the throat. This may be associated with gastro-oesophageal reflux. When a well baby presents with vomiting after every feed, one must know whether there is blood in the vomitus: it would point to a hiatus hernia or reflux. Numerous infections present as vomiting. The principle ones are otitis media, urinary tract infection, whooping cough, 'winter vomiting disease', meningitis and gastroenteritis. It is useful to know whether any other child in the family is poorly with vomiting. With regard to whooping cough, the fact that the vomiting is the result of coughing may only be elicited on careful questioning. The virus infection termed 'winter vomiting' occurs in well babies with no fever or diarrhoea. Vomiting may precede diarrhoea in gastroenteritis. Vomiting may be an early symptom of coeliac disease or adrenocortical hyperplasia.

Vomiting may be due to obstruction in the alimentary tract, including intussusception and strangulated hernia.

Vomiting may be the side-effect of drugs.

A complaint that the baby is constantly vomiting may be one of the early indications of the child abuse syndrome.

Vomiting after infancy

Causes of vomiting after infancy include, in particular, infections (especially otitis media, tonsillitis, urinary tract infection, meningitis, whooping cough and gastroenteritis), migraine and the periodic syndrome, travel sickness, intestinal obstruction, appendicitis and the effect of drugs and excessive or unusual food intake. Do not forget the possibility of a cerebral tumour.

Disposal (acute cases)

When in doubt the child has to be admitted. If he is sent home, the family doctor is spoken to on the telephone, and the child must be seen again next day.

In some cases re-examination after an hour or so may help.

Haematemesis

Haematemesis is a rare symptom in children. The new baby may swallow blood from his mother's cracked nipple. (For the test to determine whether the blood is the mother's or the baby's, see p. 119.) Older children may vomit blood after epistaxis, or in association with acute tonsillitis, or as a result of oesophageal varices or gastric ulceration from aspirins. Other causes are hiatus hernia and reflux, blood diseases, pyloric stenosis (rarely) and drugs other than aspirins.

Diarrhoea

Several conditions are often confused with gastroenteritis. Many doctors have failed to realize that a fully breast-fed baby has loose stools which are often bright green, explosive, contain mucus and curds (soap plaques), and may be very frequent—up to 24 in 24 hours. Some confuse the loose, green, starvation stools of an underfed baby with gastroenteritis. Babies with Hirschsprung's disease may present with diarrhoea and vomiting. Necrotizing enterocolitis occurs especially in low birth-weight babies who are bottle fed: they have fever, shock, diarrhoea, vomiting and abdominal distension. Carbohydrate intolerance is commonly associated with diarrhoea. Some children with acute appendicitis, peritonitis and intussusception have diarrhoea. Toddlers, aged twelve months to two or three years, sometimes have very loose stools, though well and thriving: the condition is termed the irritable colon syndrome, or 'toddler diarrhoea'. It has to be distinguished from the various diseases associated with steatorrhoea. One has seen many children treated by antidiarrhoea medicines for incontinence of faeces and liquid stools leaking out of the anus due to gross constipation. At any age ulcerative colitis may occur: blood and mucus may not appear in the stool for some months after the first attack of diarrhoea. Many medicines, such as penicillin by mouth, cause diarrhoea.

Diarrhoea is *not* due to teething.

When a child with gastroenteritis is referred to the casualty doctor or family doctor, an important decision has to be made: namely whether he is to be allowed to go home, or whether hospital treatment is required. The first essential is to decide how ill the child is: if he is ill he should be admitted. The next essential is to assess the degree of dehydration, if any.

Dehydration can be very rapid in a baby or young child. It is assessed as follows:

> Mild dehydration (< 5%)—good general condition and some loss of skin turgor.
>
> Moderate (5%)—looks ill with a dry mouth but no peripheral circulatory failure.
>
> Severe (10%)—signs of peripheral circulatory failure and gross dehydration.
>
> Over (10%)—the child is severely shocked and moribund.

When a baby is overweight it is difficult to assess the dehydration. An overweight baby may have severe acidosis and dehydration without apparent loss of tissue turgor, because fatty tissue is largely water-free. Better signs of dehydration in a fat baby are a dry mouth, a sunken fontanelle and sunken eyes. Overventilation suggests hypernatraemic acidosis and one must look for an associated infection, such as otitis media, urinary tract infection or septicaemia.

If a baby's general condition is good and there is only slight loss of tissue turgor, a rectal swab is taken and he is taken off all food for 24 hours (not more) and given an oral electrolyte solution. This can be made with Electrosol tablets (eight in a litre of water) or by using Dioralyte sachets. Dioralyte contains dextrose in addition to sodium and potassium chloride and sodium bicarbonate, and a sachet is made up to 200 ml with water.

An infant is given 150–200 ml per kg per 24 hours of this solution, but not exceeding 1·5 l. It replaces all milk and other feeds. This should not be given for more than 48 hours.

An older child is given 1–3 l in the 24 hours. The water should be tepid, for iced water increases peristalsis. Antibiotics are not given. Even if Sonne dysentery is diagnosed, they are not given, because they prolong the carrier state; the same applies to a salmonella infection. It is futile to prescribe kaolin. Diphenoxylate (Lomotil) should not be prescribed. Do not give metoclopramide or prochlorperazine.

If the child is sent home, the family doctor is spoken to, and if necessary asked to see the baby later in the day. *The parents are told that if there is any deterioration in his condition he must be brought to the hospital immediately.* He must certainly be seen next day.

If the child is ill with loss of tissue turgor and a depressed fontanelle, he must be admitted. Blood is taken for culture, blood urea and electrolytes and an intravenous line is set up with 0·45% sodium chloride in 4·8% dextrose. Give 25 ml per kg as fast as the drip will run before admitting the child. If the baby is profoundly shocked give 10 ml per kg plasma by push before attempting replacement of the deficit.

For deficit replacement, 5% dehydration will need 50 ml per kg and 10% dehydration will need 100 ml per kg. Maintenance is worked out as 2 ml per kg of body weight. The procedure is summarized below:

```
0–1 h ──────→ 4 h ──────→ 12 h ──────→      24 h
⅓ replacement ⅓ replacement ⅓ replacement
        +             +              maintenance
     maintenance   maintenance       +
        +          on-going losses
                on-going losses
```

The doctor should anticipate the development of convulsions if there is hypertonic dehydration.

Gastroenteritis in a baby or young child must be treated with caution because he can deteriorate with extreme rapidity, collapse and die.

Further reading

FRASER G.C. & WILKINSON A.W. Neonatal Hirschsprung's disease. *Br. Med. J.* 1967; ii:7.

SANTULLI T.V. *et al.* Acute necrotizing enterocolitis in infancy. *Pediatrics* 1975; **55**:376

Blood in the stool

When a baby passes blood in the stool (or vomits blood) in the first two or three days, one must know whether it is the baby's blood or the mother's blood. If necessary the stool or vomitus is filtered, and to the pink solution four or five drops of N/5 NaOH are added: if it is the baby's blood the solution remains pink because the fetal haemoglobin is more resistent to alkali, but if it is the mother's blood, the colour changes to yellow. If it is the baby's blood the baby's general condition and haemoglobin is watched. A transfusion may be necessary.

If a rectal thermometer has been used, the bleeding may be due to that.

After the newborn period the commonest causes are constipation, dysentery or salmonella infection, intussusception or ulcerative colitis. Blood from a Meckel's diverticulum is partly red and partly black. Blood may also come from a duplication of the intestine, a polyp, a foreign body or blood disease. Aspirin can cause bleeding.

Blood in the stool has to be distinguished from staining by diazepam syrup, viprynium or red gelatin.

Further reading

RUTHERFORD R.B. Meckel's diverticulum. *Surgery* 1966; **59**:618.

Rectal prolapse

Rectal prolapse is a relatively common complication of fibrocystic disease of the pancreas and of meningomyelocele. In otherwise normal children it is usually a self-limiting condition, regressing as the child grows. The parents should be shown how to replace the bowel, by elevating the buttocks, inserting a finger previously covered with tissue paper into the lumen of the protruding mass, and pushing it back into the rectum.

The skin

Nappy rash

There are four principle forms of nappy rash:

1 *The common 'ammonia dermatitis'*. This avoids the folds of the groin. It is a diffuse erythema, often with some crusting. It is now known that this is not due to irritation by ammonia but to irritation of the skin by prolonged contact with a wet nappy.

It follows that the longer the wet nappy is left in contact with the skin, the greater the likelihood of the nappy rash. The doctor must see that the mother has enough nappies (three or four dozen) to change them sufficiently frequently. A polypropylene-type nappy (e.g. Marathon, Drinap) next to the skin allows the urine to pass through to the outside (to be caught by a Terry-towel-type nappy) leaving the part next to the skin dry. Leaving the baby with the buttocks exposed to the air will clear many cases. Numerous preparations will clear the rash such as Zinc ointment B.P. or Boots E.45. Another is the N.F. hydrocortisone and clioquinol ointment. *No corticosteroid should be used for more than a week* because of the risk of damage to the skin.

It is futile to give medicine on the assumption that there is 'something wrong with the urine'.

2 *Monilial dermatitis*. This consists of isolated vesicles. There may be monilial stomatitis, or the mother may have monilial infection in the vagina. The dermatitis is treated by nyastatin cream. When a nappy rash has persisted for over ten to fourteen days, despite treatment, it is likely to be due to being secondarily infected by monilia. It is best treated by Ung. Nystaform H.C.

3 *Seborrhoeic (eczematous) dermatitis*. This is a diffuse, shiny, red rash involving the creases also. It is treated by the N.F. hydrocortisone and clioquinol ointment, or the hydrocortisone and nystatin cream, Ung. Nystaform H.C.

4 *Psoriasiform dermatitis*. Psoriasiform lesions spread from the nappy area to the body, face and limbs. This is related to psoriasis in adults. It is treated by 1% hydrocortisone, for a few days only, or, as there is commonly an associated moniliar infection, by Ung. Nystaform H.C.

Scabies and papular urticaria

It is common that children are brought with itchy rashes, particularly over a holiday period when family doctors may be less easily available.

The two which can cause most confusion in diagnosis are scabies and papular urticaria.

Scabies

In many cases the lesions have been scratched and secondarily infected and unless an underlying scabies infection is suspected, treatment of the secondary infection will not be effective.

The sites of the burrows and the sites of the sensitivity rash which can be part of the clinical picture vary in babies and very young children from that in adults. There may be a linear quality to the lesions in babies.

quality to the lesions in babies.

The sites of the burrows in children are the:

> Hands (sides and backs of the fingers), the wrists and the palms in the very young child.
>
> Elbows.
>
> Anterior axillary folds.
>
> Anterior trunk (in babies).
>
> Pubic region.
>
> Feet (soles in babies).
>
> Head and scalp which may be involved in children under two.

The sites of the sensitivity rash are the:

> Forearms.
>
> Upper arms.
>
> Trunk.
>
> Axillary folds.
>
> Legs ⎫
> Neck ⎪
> Face ⎬ in babies.
> Scalp ⎭

The main differential diagnoses in scabies in children are:

> Impetigo.

Papular urticaria
Animal scabies.
Atopic eczema.
Seborrhoeic eczema.
Napkin 'psoriasis'
Chicken-pox.

If possible the acarus should be isolated from a burrow but the child may have to be treated on a clinical diagnosis.

Treatment

Various preparations are effective, e.g. benzyl benzoate, 1% gamma benzene hexachloride (Lorexane) as a cream or lotion) or monosulfiram lotion (Tetmosol).

Lorexane is less irritating than the benzyl benzoate and should be used in young babies.

The child is given a bath, dried and the appropriate lotion applied *all over the body*, including the hands and feet but avoiding the eyes. The application of the lotion is repeated in 24 hours, then 24 hours later the child is given another bath and the sheets are washed. Monosulfiram lotion is diluted with two to three parts of water just before use and can be repeated daily for two to three days after a hot bath. A soothing application such as Boots E.45 may be needed after the treatment and a few children may develop sensitivity reactions to the applications.

The other members of the household should be treated too.

It is important to remember that irritation may persist for a week or two after treatment and this does not mean that repeated applications should be made.

Papular urticaria

(See also the section on vesicular eruptions, p. 124.)

This is commonly due to sensitivity to insect bites; the insects may be fleas from the pet dog or cat or other animals, bugs, midges, mosquitoes, etc.

The lesions occur in crops and tend to be grouped. *The*

main points of difference between scabies and papular urticaria are: in scabies adults are also affected; the lesions are more symmetrical than in papular urticaria; the hands and feet are involved frequently in scabies but seldom in papular urticaria; and there are burrows present and the lesions persist without treatment.

Treatment

The pet animals and their bedding have to be treated for their fleas. Insect repellant must be used if the urticaria is due to midges, etc.

Monosulfiram (Tetmosol) (see above) is also effective against fleas, lice and ticks.

An antihistamine may be necessary for a day or two to relieve itching.

Generalized urticaria

(See also the section on oedema of the eyelids, p. 81.)

Urticaria may be part of the picture of angioneurotic oedema or may occur without face and joint swellings.

Urticaria may be due to allergy to foodstuffs, and the particular foodstuff responsible may be known to the parents. Recent work has indicated that urticaria is often caused by tartrazine-containing foods and drugs. Tartrazine is an azo-dye used as a colouring agent in many foods and drugs, such as orange-squash, smoked fish, and various antihistamines.

The author has seen several children with urticaria treated with tartrazine-containing antihistamines so that the child is often made worse, especially if the mother is told to increase the dose when the rash gets worse.

Another cause of urticaria can be sodium benzoate which is used as a preservative in pickles, sauces, instant coffee and other foods and drinks.

Urticaria is also caused by penicillin, aspirin, barbiturates, antitoxins, iodine-containing contrast media and brewers' yeast.

Antihistamines are often helpful. Piriton (chlorpheniramine) tablets and syrup are now free from tartrazine and another which is free is Dimotane (brompheniramine).

In a particularly severe acute case hydrocortisone succinate may be necessary initially.

If you are presented with a child with urticaria, take a careful history, especially with regard to drugs, because frequently one finds that stopping them is the answer.

Some other vesicular eruptions

(See also the section on scabies and papular urticaria, pp. 121 and 122.)

Herpetic whitlow on the finger. These are seen quite commonly in young children. Herpes presents as 'grouped vesicles on an inflamed base'. The vesicles may become confluent in a few days. Apart from keeping the part clean, *no treatment is required. It should not be incised.* It takes about ten days to heal. The infection may have originated from another member of the family (e.g. with a 'cold sore'), or from a herpetic stomatitis. Remember that dummies are often shared by siblings and spread the infection.

'Hand, foot and mouth' disease

(See also p. 135).

This is due to the coxsackie virus: there are vesicles on the soles of the feet and the palms of the hands, as well as lesions in the mouth. No treatment is needed.

Chicken-pox

The lesions come in three to five successive crops over a period of two to seven days. They are itchy. Most are on the skin of the trunk but there may be ulcerating vesicles in the mouth. Differential diagnosis is generalized herpes infection, vaccinia, impetigo, drug eruptions, 'hand, foot and mouth' disease, papular urticaria and dermatitis herpetiformis.

Normally no local treatment is required, but itching can be relieved somewhat by a calamine lotion.

All scars following chicken-pox (and smallpox) are due to scratching with resultant infection.

Molluscum contagiosum

This is a viral infection. There are small papules which are umbilicated and pearly colour in appearance. They tend to be grouped. Treatment is to pierce the lesion with a pointed stick dipped in 1% phenol. If there are large numbers the dermatologist should see the child.

Bullous eruptions

These are usually due to scalds, urticaria, impetigo, pemphigus and drugs, particularly iodides, penicillin, sulphonamides, salicylates, nitrazepam, thiazide diuretics and tricyclic antidepressants. When the skin is peeling off over large areas leaving a 'scalded' appearance, it is usually a toxic epidermal necrolysis. This may be infective in origin (staphylococcal) but is often due to drugs such as sulphonamide, phenytoin or barbiturates. Paraffin can also give extensive epidermal necrolysis.

Exfoliative dermatitis

This may be caused by phenytoin, barbiturates, carbamezapine, sulphonamides, opiates, gold salts, chloroquine, penicillin, phenothiazines and streptomycin. There may be peeling of the hands and feet after a streptococcal infection.

Impetigo

A small area may clear with a simple antiseptic cream such as chlorhexidine. Local antibiotics are potentially hazardous and fucidin cream very rapidly produces resistant staphylococci. If the infected area is more extensive, systemic antibiotics are the method of choice e.g. phenoxymethyl penicillin if it is streptococcal, or cloxacillin if it is staphylococcal—the organism having first been cultured. *One must look for an underlying scabies or pediculosis.* The child should be kept from school until it is healed.

The use of corticosteroid ointment which has been prescribed or just used by the parent can result in the original lesions spreading and multiplying, often producing an appearance unlike impetigo. *It is important to ask about any treatment* which has already been given.

Boils

Simple boils are left to nature, unless it becomes obviously necessary to incise them. Antibiotics are not useful. If one is incised, a swab should be taken. A boil should not be covered up by strapping, for that may spread the infection. The skin around the boil is cleaned six to eight times a day with 3% chlorhexidine cream. For recurrent boils, the nose should be swabbed for staphylococci and if necessary treated by an appropriate antibiotic. The skin is kept as clean as possible, and hexachlorophane soap may be used. The urine is checked for sugar. There may be a reservoir of staphylococci in another member of the family (e.g. a chronic antrum infection) and this must be treated.

Abscesses should be incised in skin creases as far as possible.

Pediculosis capitis (nits)

In any impetiginous lesion of the scalp make sure that there is not an underlying pediculosis.

Gamma benzene hexachloride (Lorexane) is used, two applications to the scalp at intervals of five days. If this does not cure the condition, 0·5% malathion lotion (Prioderm) is rubbed into the scalp, avoiding the eyes. The hair is left to dry and left unwashed for 12 hours. It is then shampooed and combed with a fine-tooth comb while wet. The routine is repeated in a week. The substance is flammable and poisonous. *It should be applied only by a nurse,* and not by the parents. The nurse should wear rubber gloves.

The rest of the family should be treated.

Purpura

Purpura *in the newborn* may be due to the trauma of delivery: it is normal to find some petechial haemorrhages on the skin, particularly on the presenting part, and about a quarter of all babies have small retinal haemorrhages. Neonatal thrombocytopenic purpura is usually acquired from the mother via a platelet agglutinin or an autoimmune process: it recovers without treatment within two or three months. Thrombocytopenic purpura may be due to the cytomegalovirus or rubella, or result from renal vein thrombosis. It may be due to the mother taking certain drugs in pregnancy, notably chlorothiazide or quinine. Purpura sometimes occurs in blood group incompatibility, in septicaemia, in the presence of a giant naevus, or in toxoplasmosis. One has several times seen mongolian pigmentation in the sacral area of the buttocks and front of the ankles confused with purpura.

After the new born period the causes of purpura are numerous. The finding of only one or two purpuric spots in an acutely unwell child should suggest a meningococcal infection and treatment is urgent (see the sections on coma and convulsions, pp. 38 and 41).

Apart from trauma, the other main causes are anaphylactoid purpura, idiopathic thrombocytopenic purpura, other blood diseases, and drugs, of which over 400 are known to be causes.

In anaphylactoid purpura there are commonly petechiae on the extensor surface of the limbs and around the buttocks, often with abdominal pain and joint effusion. All blood tests are negative, as is the capillary fragility, whereas in thrombocytopenic purpura the low platelet count, the prolonged bleeding time and the abnormal capillary fragility are distinguishing features.

Sunburn

Mild sunburn will settle in a day or two without treatment. Calamine lotion may make the patient more comfortable. Severe sunburn and blistering has to be treated as an ordinary burn (see p. 55).

When faced with a child with severe sunburn, one must remember the possibility that the child has been rendered *photosensitive by drugs*. The worst offender is the tetracycline group, especially demeclocycline (Ledermycin). Photosensitivity due to this drug may last for many weeks, until the drug is eliminated from the skin, and the parents must therefore be warned to keep the child out of the sun, covering the body as much as possible, including the hands, protecting the face with a large hat and with the application of mexenone (Uvistat) cream. The parents must be told the cause, and the family doctor informed.

Other drugs which cause photosensitivity reactions include the phenothiazine and tranquillizing groups, the thiazide diuretics, sulphonamides, antihistamines, griseofulvin, nalidixic acid, antiemetics, barbiturates, carbamazepine, diphenoxylate, sulphonamides and viprynium.

Because local antihistamine preparations can cause allergic dermatitis as well as photosensitivity, in the treatment of sunburn calamine lotion B.P. is preferable to Caladryl which contains diphenhydramine hydrochloride and camphor as additives.

Remember that a number of preparations used to protect the skin from the sun can actually sensitize it to light, e.g. oil of bergamot in proprietary sun creams and oils, and rarely, mexenone (Uvistat).

Erythema nodosum

Red indurated areas are found usually on the front of the lower legs. If originally only one side is affected, it may be difficult to differentiate it from cellutitis.

Tuberculosis is the most common cause in developing countries, but is rare in Great Britain. It may follow a streptococcal infection and be a symptom of sarcoid; or it may in a child who is tuberculin positive, appear in the recovery stage of measles. It may also be caused by drugs, sulphonamides, penicillin, barbiturates, bromides, iodides, salicylates and thiouracil.

No local treatment is required but the child should be seen by a paediatrician.

Other skin conditions

A 'lump' in the upper arm following triple immunization is of no importance and requires no treatment. It is a granuloma due to the aluminium hydroxide in the injection and lasts a few weeks.

An inflamed area (later with discharge) following BCG, normally requires no treatment.

Cracks behind the ears

These clear quickly with 1% hydrocortisone cream. It should not be used for more than a week. Cracking behind the ears may occasionally be the cause of cervical abscess.

Chilblains

There is no specific treatment. An effort should be made to prevent them by keeping the hands and feet warm.

Mitten injury

If the tips of only one or two fingers are swollen or discoloured in a baby, remember that it might be a 'mitten injury' (see p. 97).

Fore-foot eczema

This is common in eight- to twelve-year-olds in hot weather. There is shiny, erythematous, fissured skin on the sole of the fore-foot and toes. It is thought to be caused by wearing socks of man-made fibres and shoes with PVC linings. It is *not*

contact dermatitis or eczema and the toe webs are clear. It
may be akin to prickly heat. Pure cotton or wool socks should
be worn and leather shoes with cork insoles. Whenever possible the child should wear open sandals or go bare foot. With
this, most cases settle but occasionally Lassar's paste in 2%
coal tar may help.

Other causes of pruritus

There are many important causes of pruritus, other than those
mentioned in the above section. The infant's skin may be sensitive to nylon or wool pants, to the dye in pants, to the deter-
gent used for washing them, to the nappy liners, or to the
elastic of the nappy holder. Infants are commonly sensitive to
wool or nylon in the vest or other clothes and the itching rash
is difficult to distinguish from a sweat rash.

Other skin conditions causing pruritus include ringworm,
psoriasis, threadworms (causing pruritus ani or vulvae), pity-
riasis, rosea, dermatitis and herpetiformis. There is commonly
itching in connnection with hyposensitization, injections and
sometimes at the site of immunization.

Drugs which may cause pruritus include aminophylline,
antibiotics, antihistamines, antisena, antiepileptic drugs, aspirin, chloral, clonidine, chloroquine, codeine, dichloral-
phenazone, diphenozylate, gold, griseofulvin, imipramine,
indomethacin, isoniazid, meprobamate, methimazole, nalidixic
acid, phenothiazine, piperazine and tetanus toxoid.

Oedema

Oedema of the *newborn* may be due to haemolytic disease or
maternal diabetes. It results also from cold injury. It may
follow positive-pressure ventilation.

In *later infancy* it can result from nephritis, the nephrotic
syndrome and hypoproteinaemia (due to malnutrition, fibrocystic disease to the pancreas, burns, extensive suppuration or
oozing eczema). Heart failure or severe anaemia as causes are
rare in children.

Angioneurotic oedema can be due to a large number of causes (see also the section on urticaria, p. 122). Aspirin may produce general oedema as well as local swelling of the face, urticaria and joint swellings.

General oedema can result from excess sodium or fluid in intravenous therapy.

Slight oedema may occur for a few days on commencing treatment for diabetes mellitus.

Oedema of the sternum is often an early feature of mumps.

Oedema of an arm is common in normal babies. The mother is horrified when on picking the baby out of the cot in the morning, she finds that an arm is cold, blue and oedematous. It is probably due to the arm being uncovered at night when it is cold. It settles in a few hours.

For oedema of the eyelids and conjunctiva, see p. 81.

When a female baby has oedema of the legs, Turner's syndrome is a likely diagnosis.

Oedema of the scrotum may be due to irritation by detergents in the clothes or nappy, to extravasation of urine if there is urethral obstruction, or to superficial cellulitis.

Swelling of the face

Apart from trauma, the main causes of facial swelling are parotitis, tumour of the parotid, dental abscess and osteitis. Though parotitis is usually due to mumps, it can be the so-called 'recurrent parotitis', in which the child has recurrent episodes of painful parotid swelling lasting a day or more and usually ceasing in adolescence. No treatment is available. A stone in the parotid duct is rare in children. A parotid swelling may be a side-effect of potassium iodide or clonazepam.

If there is an abscess in the pre-auricular region, look carefully for a congenital dermal sinus on or near the ear.

A calculus in the duct of a submandibular gland may occur in childhood and may result in a painful swelling under the jaw. The orifice of the duct may be seen to be bulging and sometimes pus can be extruded. X-ray may help in the diagnosis.

Further reading

MAYNARD J.D. Recurrent parotid swelling. *Brit. J. Surg.* 1965; **52**:784.

Headache and neurological symptoms

Most children sooner or later have a headache. The commonest cause with which they are seen in Casualty is migraine, or any of the ordinary infections. Headache may arise from the ear or a tooth, or be a side-effect of a drug. The onset of headache with vomiting *must* be taken seriously and the possibility of meningitis considered.

Many children who have headache after a minor head injury are found to have an infection, e.g. in an ear, but all children with headache after an injury must be examined fully and followed up.

Some children have headache when they have a low blood sugar for any reason, e.g. missing a meal or being starved for an anaesthetic. Hunger can precipitate an attack of migraine in some children.

A child presenting with his first attack of migraine may be difficult to diagnose with certainty. The acute occipital headache is much more likely to be due to organic disease than a frontal one, and if the onset has been sudden, one would think first of a subarachnoid haemorrhage. Various features are said to distinguish the headache of increased intracranial pressure from other headaches (for instance, the effect of posture in the former), but those features are not reliable. Examination of the optic fundi and estimation of the blood pressure are essentials in making a diagnosis. *No such child should be sent home without being seen by a senior doctor and most will need to be admitted.*

Trismus

Trismus may be due to mumps, a dental abscess, a peritonsillar abscess, an unerupted tooth or osteitis. It may result from a fracture or dislocation of the jaw. It is often a feature of feature of serum sickness and it may be a side-effect of drugs, serum sickness and it may be a side-effect of drugs, such as the phenothiazine and other tranquillizing drugs, antihistamines, metoclopramide or an overdose of strychnine. It is a feature of tetanus or rabies.

Vertigo

Vertigo, apart from that at the onset of a faint, is an unusual symptom in childhood. It may occur as 'epidemic vertigo' or 'vestibular neuronitis', probably due to a virus infection, with nausea, vomiting and nystagmus. It may be 'benign paroxysmal vertigo', occurring especially in the pre-school child, with attacks of instantaneous onset, causing the child to be terrified, to cling to his mother, and to be ataxic: it lasts for a minute or two, and may be confused with epilepsy. Vertigo may be a feature of migraine, of hypoglycaemia, of a cerebral tumour, or a side-effect of one of numerous drugs, such as antihistamines, antiepileptic drugs, tranquillizing drugs, clonidine, fenfluramine, gentamicin, indomethacin, isoniazid, nalidixic acid, sulphonamides and salicylates.

Ataxia

The acute onset of ataxia may be due to a virus encephalitis, a cerebral space-occupying lesion, solvent-sniffing, or to any of numerous drugs, such as antiepileptics and diazepam. Children being treated for threadworms may present with ataxia due to piperazine.

Involuntary movements

The acute onset of involuntary movements, such as torsion spasm, suggests the side-effect of a drug, such as metoclopramide, tranquillizing drugs, antihistamines, fenfluramine, cephalosporins, haloperidol, phenytoin or ethosuccimide.

Tremors may be caused by aminophylline and hiccoughs by ethosuccimide.

Confusion

Sudden confusion occurs in hypoglycaemia, migraine, temporal lobe epilepsy or heat stroke. It may be the side-effect of numerous drugs and poisons, such as alcohol, tranquillizing drugs, antiepileptics, antihistamines, fenfluramine, hyoscine, indomethacin, nitrofurantoin and solvent-sniffing.

Drowsiness

The onset of drowsiness in an ill child *must* be taken seriously. It may be an early symptom of any infection, including meningitis. It may be due to diabetes, renal or hepatic failure, dehydration or drugs (such as those which cause confusion).

Acute neck stiffness

Though neck stiffness is a major feature of meningism, there is frequently no neck stiffness in infants with pyogenic meningitis. In neck stiffness of meningitis or meningism, the stiffness is only on flexion of the neck, and is associated with pain in the erector spinae muscles in the lumbar region when the head is flexed.

Neck stiffness may be due to injury, and it may not be easy to elicit the relevant history from a boy who prefers to conceal some of his actions. It may be due to osteitis in the cervical vertebrae.

Neck stiffness in the morning is a characteristic feature of rheumatoid arthritis. Neck stiffness with pain on rotation and tenderness on pressure, the so-called 'rheumatic' stiff neck, may be due to a virus infection, or to posture in sleep.

Neck stiffness may result from cervical adenitis or a retropharyngeal abscess. It may be due to drugs such as metoclopromide and the tranquillizers.

X-rays of the cervical spine should be done with the neck extended as well as flexed. If this is not done there may be an appearance which suggests a subluxation (see Fig. 10).

Nystagmus

By far the commonest cause of nystagmus in a baby or toddler is a defect of vision. Rarely nystagmus is congenital: it is usual in albinism and is a feature of spasmus nutans. It occurs in cerebellar and cerebellar tract lesions. It may be caused by antiepileptic drugs, salicylates, colistin and diphenoxylate.

Further reading

DUNN D.W. & SNYDER H. Benign paroxysmal vertigo of childhood. *Am. J. Dis. Child.* 1976; **130**:1099.

Symptoms in the ear, nose and throat

Choanal atresia is manifested at birth by cyanosis and dyspnoea when the mouth is shut; as soon as the baby opens the mouth he breathes normally. The treatment consists of the insertion of an airway through the mouth, followed by elective surgery.

Stomatitis is commonly seen in a casualty department. It is frequently due to herpes, coxsackie or other viruses. There may also be vesicles on hands and feet ('hand, foot and mouth' disease). The virus infections have a self-limiting course of about ten days, and no specific treatment helps; antibiotics are useless. They do not need idoxuridine. Severe cases in which the child is unable to take fluids should be admitted, but normally the child can go home. The fluid intake must be maintained. If the child is old enough he should use a drinking straw. Cold drinks and food such as ice-cream are most comfortable. The mother must be told that the condition usually lasts about ten days and that if she finds it impossible to get the child to drink admission will be arranged. *Do not admit him near children who are on immuno-suppressive therapy*.

The other common cause of a stomatitis is a thrush infection due to monilia. This is common in babies and may be associated with a napkin rash (see also p. 120). It can also occur in older children who have been on antibiotics. The lesions are creamy-white and are on the tongue and buccal mucosa. They cannot easily be removed by a swab. Treatment is with Nystatin, 100 000 units in 1 ml. One ml is put on to the tongue four times daily between feeds. An associated napkin rash must be treated. Occasionally it may be resistant to nystatin and miconazole (Daktarin gel) is then used.

Vincent's infection is uncommon in children. In doubtful cases a smear should be made.

Gingivitis and stomatitis may be due to drugs, e.g. phenytoin, and certain blood diseases such as scurvy. It may be part of the Stevens-Johnson syndrome in which there is a severe stomatitis associated with a rash in a poorly, feverish child. In many cases the cause is not found but one of the drugs known to cause it is cotrimoxazole (Septrin).

When a child is found to have *acute tonsillitis,* ideally a swab should be taken and if next day haemolytic streptococci have been cultured, oral penicillin is given for a full ten day course. If it is given for less, there is a bigger relapse rate. Many throat infections are viral and it is impossible to differentiate them clinically from streptococcal infections.

Membrane on the tonsil. The commonest cause in this country is infectious mononucleosis, but in developing countries it is still diphtheria. Do not be confused by the closely similar 'membrane' immediately following tonsillectomy.

Acute otitis media is usually due to the haemolytic streptococcus and often to the haemophilus influenzae. In the past, one injection of Triplopen followed by 125 mg of phenoxymethyl penicillin six hourly for ten days seemed to be satisfactory, but a controlled trial showed that amoxycillin was superior to other treatments. Cotton-wool plugs are *not* inserted, and it is futile to prescribe ear drops.

Otitis externa may be treated by cotton-wool wicks soaked in ichthyol and glycerin daily after mopping out the discharge. An underlying otitis media is treated as above. Some favour the use of Locorten-Vioform ear drops (quinoline and corticosteroid) or aluminium acetate ear drops (N.F.).

The acute development of *stridor* is a serious condition and

mistakes due to overconfidence in its management have frequently led to disaster. The danger lies in the way in which
small children with apparently slight stridor may rapidly
become worse and develop serious respiratory obstruction. *A
child with acute stridor of recent onset should be admitted.* The
cause of acute stridor is usually acute laryngo-tracheo-
bronchitis, but it may be epiglottitis or a foreign body.
Laryngo-tracheo-bronchitis can easily be confused with acute
asthma, but if the child has asthma, there is likely to be a
history of a previous attack or of eczema, and on auscultation
of the chest there should be high-pitched rhonchi, but the
distinction can be difficult.

Acute laryngo-tracheo-bronchitis, like asthma, commonly follows a cold. *Acute epiglottitis* which is usually due to haemophilus influenzae, is more serious: it occurs particularly in the
two- to four-year-old group. After a mild upper respiratory
tract infection the child becomes ill, with increasing dyspnoea,
a low-pitched stridor, and a low-pitched expiratory rattle,
often with drooling and salivation. The voice may be muffled
rather than hoarse. As a rough guide, if the voice is hoarse and
weak, the glottis is involved. If the voice is normal while there
is severe stridor and dyspnoea, the obstruction is tracheal or
subglottic. If there is a high pitched stridor which is both
inspiratory and expiratory, there is severe glottic obstruction.
A low pitched stridor is of supraglottic origin. Stridor with a
brassy cough suggests tracheal obstruction.

*Neither the family doctor nor the casualty doctor should examine
the throat; a throat examination might cause cardiac and respiratory
arrest. The child should be seen immediately by the paediatrician
and the ear, nose and throat specialist.*

The problem of the foreign body in the larynx is discussed
on p. 51. *A retropharyngeal abscess* causes difficulty in breathing, difficulty in swallowing, fever and head retraction. A lateral X-ray of the neck will show the abscess. Examination of
the throat is better left to the ear, nose and throat expert if the
obstruction is marked; otherwise it is said that the swelling
can be felt in the pharynx by the examining finger.

Epistaxis usually begins spontaneously from a vein in the septum. It may result from picking the nose or from a foreign body or a polyp, and it is an occasional result of rhinitis in a respiratory infection. It occurs in whooping cough, blood diseases and hypertension.

Most epistaxis arises from the anterior part of the septum, and can therefore be controlled by appropriate pressure on the nose. The nose is firmly compressed by the thumb in such a way that the anterior part of the septum is included in the pressure. This pressure is maintained for ten minutes, the doctor resisting the temptation to keep releasing the pressure in order to determine whether the bleeding has ceased. One wants a firm thrombus to form, and takes into account the normal bleeding time.

If this fails, the help of the ear, nose and throat specialist should be sought. Very rarely the nose may have to be packed. Calgitex is gauze with sodium alginate and sticks less than plain gauze.

The possibility of a blood disease has to be considered when the bleeding is not stopped by the ordinary methods. For recurrent epistaxis, the child is referred to the ear, nose and throat specialist in the out-patient department for cauterizing the source of bleeding, if one is found.

Further reading

BRITISH MEDICAL JOURNAL Leading article: antibiotics for otitis media. 1976; 4:1407.

Some respiratory symptoms

In the newborn baby dyspnoea may be due to the respiratory distress syndrome, pneumothorax, mediastinal emphysema, diaphragmatic hernia or massive aspiration of amniotic fluid in delivery.

After the newborn period, dyspnoea, apart from the obvious causes such as pneumonia, bronchiolitis or asthma, may be due to a foreign body, pneumothorax, obstructive emphysema, pleural effusion, or heart failure (e.g. in paroxysmal tachycardia). Respiratory muscle paralysis in poliomyelitis or the Guillain Barré syndrome causes rapid respirations and can readily be confused with pneumonia: poor respiratory excursions may give the correct diagnosis.

Over-ventilation

Over-ventilation occurs in older children as a hysterical symptom. In babies it is a characteristic feature of hypernatraemic acidosis. It may be due to diabetic acidosis or uraemia. It is said to be an early symptom of rabies, before spasms develop.

Over-ventilation is an important sign of salicylate poisoning; it may also be caused by sulthiame, rifampicin, acetazolamide or aminophylline. It occurs in Reye's syndrome (liver failure with encephalopathy).

Wheezing

Apart from asthma (see p. 65) and acute bronchiolitis, wheezing may be due to a foreign body, bronchial obstruction by tuberculosis or tumour, a vascular ring, fibrocystic disease of the pancreas or to certain drugs, notably propranolol, aspirin and several antibiotics.

It is a serious result of burning of the respiratory passages by inhaling smoke in a burning house.

Haemoptysis

Haemoptysis is a rare symptom in children. It may be due to a foreign body, whooping cough, malignant disease, bronchiectasis or a blood disease. It must be distinguished from red sputum after the child has taken rifampicin.

Some genitourinary symptoms
Frequency of micturition

Doctors are often consulted about the toddler who is acquiring sphincter control, and who demands to be taken to the lavatory every few minutes. This is a successful attention-seeking device, particularly when his mother is determined to 'train' him.

Frequency may be due to a urinary tract infection, pelvic peritonitis or appendicitis, or to polyuria, which in turn is due to habit polydipsia, diabetes mellitus or diabetes insipidus, renal acidosis or hypercalcaemia. Frequency may be due to drugs, notably antihistamines, carbamazepine, fenfluramine and demeclocycline.

Delayed micturition in the newborn

Two-thirds of babies pass urine in the first 12 hours, a quarter in the next 12 hours, and the remainder (7%) only after 24 hours. Most of these 7% are normal, but the possible serious conditions which might cause the delay include urethral obstruction in the male (shown by a poor stream of urine with a distended bladder), a 'neurogenic bladder' due to meningomyelocele or sacral agenesis, renal agenesis or bilateral renal vein thrombosis. Hydrocolpos or labial adhesions may cause retention in the female.

Retention of urine after the newborn period

This may be an attention-seeking device—but it is unusual. It can occasionally occur in a normal toddler who has had to wait overlong to pass urine. If put into a warm bath he may be able to pass it. Retention may result from faecal impaction, obstruction by a tumour, calculus or a foreign body. It may be caused by drugs, including phenothiazines and imipramine.

Scalding on micturition

The usual cause of this is a nappy rash or soreness of the vulva. In the circumcised boy a meatal ulcer may result from a nappy rash. Scalding may result from cystitis or from drugs—notably the tricyclic antidepressants, chlordiazepoxide and isoniazid.

Haematuria

Haematuria may be the result of a blood disease, anaphylactoid purpura, trauma to the kidney, acute nephritis or pyelonephritis, Wilms' tumour, polycystic kidney, renal calculus, renal vein thrombosis, hydronephrosis, renal tuberculosis, haemorrhagic cystitis (due to the adenovirus or cyclophosphamide) or a foreign body in the bladder. It can be caused by drugs—notably sulphonamides causing crystalluria, acetazolamide, aminophylline, cyclophosphamide, phensuccimide, phenytoin, salicylates and troxidone.

Haematuria must be distinguished from beeturia (after eating beetroot) and coloration of the urine after taking blackcurrant juice, rose hip syrup, red sweets, etc.

Scrotal swelling

The usual causes are hernia, hydrocele, tumour or torsion of the testis, cysts or trauma. For torsion of the testis see p. 112.

Paraphimosis

If the paraphimosis cannot be reduced by hand the child should be admitted.

Meatal ulcer

Lignocaine ointment eases the pain on micturition. The associated nappy rash must be treated (p. 120).

Vulvovaginitis

The clear mucoid discharge from the vagina of the newborn or around puberty is normal.

A mild vulvovaginitis may respond to simple hygiene, with

daily washing and teaching the girl to wipe from vulva backwards after defaecation. A purulent vaginal discharge usually responds to penicillin systemically. Monilial infection is treated by nystatin ointment, and threadworms by viprynium. The possibility of a foreign body should be remembered and also the possibility of child abuse. When in doubt the doctor should refer the child to the gynaecologist.

Balanitis

This is usually a self-curing condition. Cool baths help the discomfort. If retraction of the foreskin has not previously occurred, it may do after the balanitis. Balanitis is not an indication for circumcision.

Further reading

JOHNSTON J.H. Abnormalities of micturition in the neonate. *Br. J. Hosp. Med.* 1976; **16**:462.
WEST C.D. Asymptomatic haematuria and proteinuria in children. *J. Pediatr.* 1976; **89**:173.

Limp and limb pains

Many children present in a casualty department with a limp. As the possible causes are numerous, diagnosis can be difficult: often in fact the limp settles down without a definite diagnosis having been made.

Take a complete history—including drugs. The child may deny any possibility of trauma: but careful questioning may reveal that the child on the previous day had taken an active part in a vigorous game in PE or is a particularly keen member of a ballet or tap-dancing class.

Limp is an important symptom in a child and must be taken seriously. Remember that discomfort in the knee may mean a lesion in the hip and vice versa. By watching the child walk it may be possible to get a good idea of the site of discomfort. Having eliminated the common causes such as a painful shoe, a plantar wart, inflamed lymph nodes in the groin, etc., one tests the range of movements in all joints, and feels the joints for heat. In addition to testing the hips for the range of abduction, rotation and extension, it is as well to examine the spinal movements. All the bones are palpated for tenderness or slight warmth. The thigh and buttocks are examined for injection marks and inflammation.

Transient synovitis of the hip is one of the common and important causes of a limp in children. It occurs particularly between the ages of 18 months and 6 years, and is more common in boys. In two-thirds of cases there is a history of a recent upper respiratory tract infection, and in one-sixth a history of possible injury. The only symptom is a limp or some discomfort around the hip or knee. The white cell count is normal and the ESR normal or slightly raised. X-ray of the hips may show no abnormality of the bones but it is important to notice if there is any measurable increase in the joint space of the affected hip. *Transient synovitis is important because some children who have it will later develop Perthes' disease of the upper femoral epiphysis.* It is thought that the increased pressure in the joint results in some interruption to the blood supply leading to avascular necrosis.

If the child has considerable pain and has marked limitation of hip movements or local tenderness, he is admitted for traction and possible aspiration of the joint. If the discomfort and physical signs are less and home conditions are satisfactory he may go home, but transport to his home must be arranged: *he must be kept at complete rest.* He is then reviewed in two days. If there is deterioration he is admitted but if the degree of limitation is lessening and he is being kept at rest he is allowed home again, and seen in a week. If when he is re-examined after this week, there is a full range of painless movements, he is allowed to bear weight. If there has been measurable increase in joint space he should be X-rayed again in six to eight weeks' time. The parents must be told that if there is any recurrence of limp or pain before that time he must be taken off his legs and seen earlier.

Some children who come with a limp already have X-ray changes in the upper femoral epiphysis consistent with a developed Perthes' disease. They are referred to the orthopaedic department.

A slipped femoral epiphysis occurs especially in the ten- to fifteen-year-old group, more often in overweight boys: it is bilateral in 20%. The symptom is a limp with little pain. The X-ray establishes the diagnosis: a lateral view is necessary.

Signs which seem to point to a lesion in a hip may be the result of psoas spasm and the underlying disease may be in the lower spine, sacro-iliac joint or pelvis.

Some children come with recurrent episodes of limp and if care is not taken they have a large amount of irradiation of the pelvis by too frequent X-rays of the hips. In such children, particularly when there is a family history of rheumatoid arthritis, blood should be taken for rheumatoid anti-nuclear factor, and 'C' reactive protein, as they may eventually turn out to have non-articular rheumatoid arthritis or ankylosing spondylitis.

Some children get joint pains following streptococcal infections and the ASO titre may be found to be raised.

There are many other conditions which may cause a limp. They include Kohler's disease of the navicular bone, arthritis, scurvy, sickle cell anaemia and osteoid osteoma. Osteomyelitis must always be considered when a child complains of bone pains and occasionally leukaemia or other blood disease may present in this way. The whole child should be examined and the temperature taken.

The most useful investigations are an X-ray, a blood count and differential count, an ESR and a throat swab.

Many of these children will need to be referred to an orthopaedic surgeon.

Further reading

ANSELL B. *Rheumatic Disorders in Childhood*. London: Butterworth & Co., 1980.
ILLINGWORTH C.M. 128 limping children. *Clin. Pediatr. Phila.* 1977; **17**: 139.
STOCK A. Transient synovitis of the hip joint in children. *Pediatrics* 1959; **24**: 1042.

Swelling of a joint: arthritis

It would not be profitable to list the dozens of causes of arthritis in children: most of them are extremely rare. In this section, however, I shall mention some of the more important causes.

Pains in the limbs of well schoolchildren are usually the so-called 'growing pains': they are non-articular, have no relationship to rheumatic fever and the ESR is normal.

When there is swelling of a joint, the first essential is to eliminate trauma as a cause. A child may deny the possibility in his mother's presence if he has been engaged in a forbidden pursuit.

Numerous infections cause arthritis. An important one because of the urgency of treatment is meningococcal septicaemia. A thorough search for petechial haemorrhages should be made, not forgetting to look at the conjunctival surface of the lower eyelid. Arthritis with petechiae should be diagnosed as meningococcal until proved otherwise.

Osteitis near a joint causes confusion, especially if there are multiple foci of osteitis—involving several joints. X-ray is unlikely to show evidence of osteitis in the first few days. An important snare for the unwary is a low or normal white cell count in staphylococcal septicaemia: this is common. *Before any treatment is given blood should be taken for blood culture and the child admitted.*

Acute rheumatic fever is now rare in the UK but it is common in developing countries. There may be the characteristic flitting polyarthritis, the pain and swelling involving first one joint and then another, the previous joint settling down: the joints involved are the elbow, wrist, knee and ankle. The hip is rarely involved and arthritis of the hip should be ascribed to another cause unless there is other good evidence of rheumatic fever. Commonly only one joint is involved: the child is *always unwell*. There may be signs of carditis. The temperature may or may not be raised, the ESR is always high unless there is heart failure, the ASO titre is virtually always high, above 200 units, and CRP is virtually always present.

Rheumatoid arthritis is usually much less acute: only one joint may be involved. The peak age of onset is two to four years, while rheumatic fever is extremely rare at that age. If a single joint is involved, it is usually the knee or ankle or occasionally the hip (see the section on limp and limb pains, p.

142). In a few there is arthritis of the proximal interphalangeal joints of the fingers. The child is not usually ill.

A highly characteristic symptom is morning stiffness, often including stiffness of the neck. There is occasionally an evanescent, salmon-pink maculo-papular rash on the trunk, lasting a few hours at a time. The ESR is normal in a third of all cases, and rarely high (i.e. rarely above 30 mm in an hour, micromethod).

Henoch-Schönelin or anaphylactoid purpura is relatively common in children. The combination of petechial haemorrhages, especially on the buttocks, joint effusion and abdominal pain readily establishes the diagnosis, but in an occasional case the joint effusion precedes other manifestations. All blood investigations are negative (including the platelet count, bleeding and clotting time and capillary fragility) and the ESR may or may not be normal. In children of appropriate ethnic groups, sickle cell anaemia may cause joint effusions.

If a child is not known to have haemophilia, the diagnosis can be missed. As in the case of any young child with joint and particularly bone pain, the possibility of leukaemic or other malignant disease should be remembered.

Several drugs may cause a joint effusion.

Appendices

Blood pressure, weight and height

Normal blood pressure (mm Hg) (50th centile).

Age in years	0	1	2–6	8	10	12
Normal blood pressure	85	95	100	105	110	115

Weight (50th centile).
(From TANNER J.M., WHITEHOUSE
R.H. & TAKAISHI M. Standard from
birth to maturity for height, weight,
etc. *Arch. Dis. Child.* 1966; **41**:613.)

Age in years	Weight (kg) M	F
0·25	5·9	5·6
0·5	7·9	6·9
0·75	9·2	8·7
1	10·2	9·7
2	12·7	12·2
3	14·7	14·3
4	16·6	16·3
5	18·5	18·3
6	20·5	20·4
7	22·6	22·6
8	25·0	25·1
9	27·5	27·7
10	30·3	31·1

Height (50th centile).

Age in years	Height (cm) M	F
1	76·3	74·2
3	94·2	93·0
5	108·3	107·2
7	120·5	119·3
9	131·6	130·6

Normal values

Haemoglobin in children (approximate values).

Age	g/100 ml
Two weeks	17·0
Four weeks	14·0
Six months	11·0
One year	11·0
Three years	11·5
Five years	12·0
Ten years	13·0

ESR (micromethod).

	mm in one hour
0–10	Normal
11–15	Doubtful, probably slightly raised
Over 15	Definitely raised

Normal ranges of capillary plasma values for children.*

		Age					
		0–4 weeks	5–11 weeks	3–11 months	1–5 years	6–10 years	11–15 years
Sodium	mmol/litre	130–140	131–141	131–141	130–140	128–141	130–143
Potassium	mmol/litre	4·1–7·0	4·0–6·0	3·5–6·0	3·5–5·6	3·4–5·2	3·5–5·2
Bicarbonate	mmol/litre	17–27	16–28	16–26	16–25	18–26	17–27
Chloride	mmol/litre	94–110	94–110	93–110	94–110	94–109	93–110
Urea	mmol/litre	2·7–5·0	2·5–8·0	2·5–7·8	2·7–6·0	2·8–6·7	2·7–6·3
Calcium	mmol/litre	1·85–2·70	2·20–2·65	2·15–2·75	2·10–2·75	2·15–2·60	2·15–2·60
Magnesium	mmol/litre	0·50–0·85	0·60–0·95	0·65–0·95	0·65–0·90	0·60–0·85	0·60–0·90
Phosphate	mmol/litre	1·40–3·10	—	1·00–2·55	1·25–2·40	1·15–2·15	0·95–2·20
Alkaline phosphatase	U/litre	40–170	—	60–190	60–170	60–190	60–170
Bilirubin	µmol/litre	†	—	—	2–22 ▼	2–24 ▼	—
Glucose‡	mmol/litre	2·0–5·5	2·7–6·3	3·5–7·0	2·8–6·8	2·8–6·8	2·8–6·8

* 5% of the normal population will lie below the lower limit and 5% above the upper limit. As determined in the Department of Chemical Pathology, Sheffield Children's Hospital.

† 342 µmol per l of bilirubin is equivalent to 20 mg per 100 ml.

‡ Normal range for values collected at random time.

▼ Improved method now in use. Normal values may be lower than stated above.

Further reading

DE LOBO E. *Children of Immigrants to Britain*. London: Hodder & Stoughton, 1978.

HARRIS F. *Paediatric Fluid Therapy*. Oxford: Blackwell Scientific Publications, 1972.

ILLINGWORTH R.S. *Common Symptoms of Disease in Children*, 7th edn. Oxford: Blackwell Scientific Publications, 1982.

JELLIFFE D.B. & STANFIELD J.B. *Diseases of Children in the Subtropics and Tropics*. London: Edward Arnold, 1978.

KRUGMAN S. & KATZ S.L. *Infectious Diseases of Children*. St. Louis: C.V. Mosby Co., 1981.

SMITH C. *The Critically Ill Child*. Chicago: W.B. Saunders & Co., 1972.

SURGICAL STAFF, HOSPITAL FOR SICK CHILDREN, TORONTO *Care of the Injured Child*. Baltimore: Williams and Wilkins, 1975.

TOULOUKIAN R. (ed.) *Pediatric Trauma*. Chichester: John Wiley & Sons, 1978.

VERBOV J. *Paediatric Dermatology*. London: William Heinemann, 1979.

Index

Principal references in heavy print

Abdominal distension **113**
Abdominal injury **76**
Abdominal pain
  acute **109**
  recurrent **110**
Abscess
  dental 78
  retropharyngeal 137
  submandibular 78
Accidents *see* road-traffic accidents
  67
Acute illness **106**
Adrenaline
  dosage 66
  eye drops 80
Amblyopia 83
Anaesthesia, local 15
Anaphylactoid purpura 127, 146
Anaphylaxis **66**
Angioneurotic oedema 130
Antibiotics, prophylactic **13**
Anxious mother 6
Appendicitis, acute **111**
Arm, oedema of 130
Arthritis **144**
Artificial respiration 62
Aspirin poisoning *see* salicylates 33,
  34
Asthma, severe **65**
Ataxia **133**
Ataxia caused by poisons 32
Attitudes to parents 5

Balanitis 142
Battered baby *see* non-accidental
  injury 16
BCG, swelling and discharge 129
Berries, poisonous 37
Bites
  dog **99**
  snake **100**

Bladder, foreign body in 54
Bleeding tooth socket 78
Blood in stool **119**
Blood pressure, normal values **147**
Blood sugar 39
Blow-out fracture of orbit 74
Blurring of vision 83
Boils **126**
Books recommended 150
Bradycardia 32
Breath-holding attacks 43
Bronchi, foreign body in 52
Brought in dead 23
Bruising
  near eye **74**
  in non-accidental injury 19, 71
  on skull 73
Bullous eruptions **125**
Burns **55**

Cardiac
  arrest **62**
  arrhythmia caused by poisons 32
Care order 22
Cephalhaematoma 73
Cervical injury, X-rays 86
Chest injuries **75**
Chicken pox **124**
Chilblains 129
Child abuse *see* non-accidental
  injury **16**
Choanal atresia 135
Choking 51
Cigarette burns 19
Cold injury **59**
Coma
  diabetic 40
  general 31, **38**, 40
  meningococcal 41
Concussion **68**
Confusion 31, 134
Conjunctiva, oedema of 80

153

Conjunctivitis 79, 80
Convulsions **41**
  breath-holding 43
  febrile 42
  following head injury 72
  hypoglycaemia 43
  infants 42
  poisons 32
  treatment 43
Coroner's Office 24
Corrosive 32
Cot death 24
Court, witness in **25**
Cricothyreotomy 51
Criminal injury **98**
Crying baby **107**

Dead or dying children **23**
Dehydration
  assessment 117
  repair 57, **117**
Dental abscess 78
Dental injury 77
Dermatitis
  monilial 120
  psoriasiform 120
  seborrhoeic 120
Dextropropoxyphene 35
Diabetes mellitus 40
Diabetic coma 39, 40
Diarrhoea **116**
Diazepam 44
Diphenoxylate ingestion 36
Diplopia 82
Distalgesic 35
Dizziness 133
Dog bites 99
Drowning 41, **60**, 134
Drowsiness 134
Drugs
  frequency of side-effects 7
  overtreatment 12
Dyspnoea 138

Ear
  cracks behind 129
  foreign body in 49
Ear, nose and throat symptoms 135
Eczema, forefoot 129

Elbow
  injury *see* limb injury 83
  pulled **93**
Electric shock, shoulder dislocation
  56
Electrolyte figures 149
Emetic, ipecacuanha 33
Endotracheal intubation 63
Enteric-coated tablets 33
Enterocolitis, necrotizing 116
Epiglottitis 137
Epilepsy **42**
Epistaxis **138**
Erythema nodosum **128**
ESR **148**
Ethistrip **45**
Evidence in court 25
Examination **7**
Excitement 31
Exfoliative dermatitis **125**
Eye
  bruising near 74
  chemical injury 79
  foreign body in 50
  general **78**
  haemorrhage in 79
  hyphema 79
  injury **78**
  iridocyclitis 80
Eyelid
  injury **78**, 79
  oedema 81

Face, swelling of **131**
Facial bones, fractures **73**
Febrile convulsions 42
Femoral epiphysis, slipped 144
Fever, unexplained **108**
Fingertip
  amputation **96**
  injury **94**
Fingers, trapped **94**
Fits *see* convulsions 41
Fluid needs 57, 117
Foreign bodies **48**
  bladder 54
  bronchi 52
  ear 49
  eye 50, 79
  inhaled 51
  larynx 51

Foreign bodies *cont.*
  nose 49
  oesophagus 53
  skin 54
  stomach 53
  tonsils 51
  trachea 52
  vagina 54
Fractures **83**
  elbow 84, 86, 88
  facial bones 131
  non-accidental injury 19, 83
  scaphoid 86
  treatment, summary of **87**
Frenum linguae 19
Frequency of micturition 140
Fungi ingestion 37

Gastric lavage 32
Genitourinary symptoms **140**
Glass in X-rays 9, 85
Glycosuria **40**
Golf-ball injury 79
Gynaecological injury **98**

Haemaccel 57
Haematemesis 116
Haematoma
  of nasal septum 75
  of scalp **73**
  subungual 96
Haematuria 141
Haemoglobin figures 148
Haemophilia 10
Haemoptysis **139**
Hallucinations, poisons 31
'Hand, foot and mouth' disease **124**
Hay fever, eye 80
Headache **132**
Head injury **68**
  admission 72
  errors in diagnosis 10
  examination 69
  history 68
  interpretation of findings 71
  investigation 70
  treatment 72
Heart failure, acute **65**
Heat stroke 57
Height figures 147

Henoch-Schönlein purpura 127, 146
Herpetic whitlow 124
Hip, transient synovitis 143
History, taking **6**
Hoarseness 137
Holidays abroad, illnesses 105
Humotet 14
Hyperglycaemia 39
  caused by salicylates 34
Hypernatraemia 41
Hyperthermia, malignant 57, 58
Hyphema 79
Hypoglycaemia **39**
  caused by alcohol 36
  caused by salicylates 34
Hypothermia 59, **60**

Illness, acute **106**
Illness after holiday abroad 105
Immersion hypothermia 60
Immigrant children **105**
Immunization
  nodule after 129
  tetanus 14
Immunoglobulin, human tetanus 14
Impetigo **125**
Infantile spasms 43
Inhaled foreign body 51
Intubation **63**
Intussusception **111**
Investigations 9
Involuntary movements 32, 133
Ipecacuanha 33
Iridocyclitis 80
Iron poisoning **35**

Jaw injury 74
Joint swelling **144**

'Kinks' 43
Knee injuries *see* limb injury 83

Laburnum 37
Lacerations **45**
Lachrymation **82**
  caused by poisons 32
Laryngoscope 51, 63

Laryngo-tracheo-bronchitis 137
Larynx, foreign body 51
Latent period after poisoning 30, 34
Lavage, gastric 32
Leishmaniasis 105, 106
Limb
  injury **83**
  pains **142**
Limp **142**
Lip laceration 48
Litigation, common causes 4
Local anaesthesia 15
Lomotil *see* diphenoxylate 36

Malaria 106
Mandible, fracture 74
Maxillo-facial injuries 73
Meatal ulcer 141
Medicines, history of drugs taken 7
Medico-legal problems 4, 5
  with fractures 85
Meibomian cyst 81
Melaena 119
Meningism 134
Meningitis 11, 134
Micturition
  delayed 140
  frequency 140
  scalding 140
Migraine 132
Mitten injury **97**
Molluscum contagiosum **125**
Monilial infection, nappy rash 120
Monteggia fracture 85
Mouth
  dry from poisons 32
  ulcers 135
Movements, involuntary 133
Munchausen syndrome 11
Mydriatic 38, **83**

Nail injuries 94
Naloxone 35, 40
Napkin rash **120**
Nasal septum injury 75
Neck injury, X-rays 86
Neck stiffness **134**
Neurological symptoms 132
Nits **126**

Non-accidental injury **16**
  Care Order 22
  child brought in dead 24
  cot death 24
  crying baby 108
  differential diagnosis 21
  fractures 19
  legal aspects 22
  limb injury 83
  management 21
  Place of Safety Order 22
  poisoning 31
  ribs fractured 20
  summary 23
  suspicious features in history 18
Nose bleed 138
  foreign body 49
  injury 74
  haematoma of septum 75
Note-keeping **5**
Nystagmus **135**

Oedema
  arm 131
  conjunctiva 80
  eyelids 81
  generalized **131**
  legs 131
  sternum 131
Oesophagus, foreign body 53
Orbit, blow-out fracture 74
Osteomyelitis 145
Otitis
  externa 136
  media 136
Over-anxious mother 6
  in non-accidental injury 11
Over-confidence **3**
Over-ventilation **139**

Pain
  abdomen **109**
  history **106**
  renal 112
Pain in knee, referred from hip 11,
  142
Papular urticaria 122
Paracetamol 34
Paraldehyde 44
Paraphimosis 141

Parotitis 131
Pediculosis capitis **126**
Penicillin sensitivity 13
Perineal injury 98
Periosteal elevation 21
Perthes' disease 143
Photophobia 82
Photosensitivity **128**
Place of Safety Order 22
Poisoning **29**
  alcohol 36
  berries 37
  centres 29
  coma 40
  corrosives 33
  dextropropoxyphene 35
  diphenoxylate 36
  Distalgesic 35
  enteric-coated capsules 33
  examination 31
  fungi 37
  gastric lavage 32
  history 30
  investigations 31
  iron 35
  laburnum 35, 37
  latent period 30, 34
  naloxone 35
  non-accidental injury 31
  paracetamol 34
  salicylates 33, 34
  treatment 32
  yew 37
Prolapse of rectum **119**
Prophylactic antibiotics **13**
Pruritus **130**
Pulled elbow **93**
Pupils
  in coma 38
  dilated 32
  with head injury 70, 71
  small 32
Purpura **127**
  anaphylactoid 127, 146
Pyloric stenosis 115
Pyrexia of unknown origin **108**

Rabies **99**, 100
Rape 98

Rectal
  examination 9
  prolapse **119**
Referred pain **11, 67**
Respiratory arrest **62**
Resuscitation 61, **62**
Retention of urine 140
Retropharyngeal abscess 137
Rheumatic fever 145
Rheumatoid arthritis 145
Rib fractures 20
Risk register, non-accidental injury
  21
Road-traffic accidents **67**
Rubber in X-ray 53
Rumination 115

Safety Order, Place of 22
Salbutamol 65
Salicylate poisoning 33, 34
  enteric-coated capsules 33
Salivation, poisoning 32
Salt, danger as emetic 33
Scabies **121**
Scalding micturition 140
Scalds **55**
Scalp
  haemorrhage **73**
  swelling in babies **73**
Scaphoid fracture 86
Scrotal swelling **141**
Sexual abuse 22, 98
Shock, treatment **68**
Shoulder dislocation, from electric
  shock 56
Sickle cell anaemia **105**
Skin conditions **120**
Skin, foreign body 55
Skull, X-rays of 70
Slipped femoral epiphysis 144
Snake bite **100**
Spin-dryer injury **92**
Steristrip 45
Sternum, oedema of 130
Stings **98**
Stitches, removal of 48
Stitching lacerations 45
Stomach, foreign body in 53
Stomach lavage 32
Stomatitis 135
Stool, blood in **119**

Stridor 136
Stye 81
Submandibular abscess 78
Subungual haematoma 96
Sunburn **128**
Sutures, time of removal 48
Synovitis of hip, transient 143

Tachycardia caused by poisons 32
Tartrazine 123
Teeth 77
  displaced 77
Teething 42
Temperature taking 9
Testis, torsion of **112**
Tetanus, immunization 14, 15
Thoracic injuries **75**
Throat, foreign body in 51
Thrush 135
Tongue, laceration 48
Tonsillar membrane 136
Tonsillitis 136
Tooth
  bleeding socket 78
  broken 77
  displaced 77
Torsion of testis 112
Torsion spasms caused by poisons
    32, 133
Trachea, foreign body in 52
Trapped fingers **94**
Treatment, discussion 12
Tremors 133
Trismus 32, **132**

Urine
  examination 9
  retention 140
Urticaria **122**, 123

Vagina
  bleeding from non-accidental
    injury 18
  discharge 141

Vagina *cont.*
  foreign body in **54**
Ventricular fibrillation 63
Vertigo **133**
Vesicular eruptions 124
Vincent's stomatitis 136
Vision, blurred 83
Vomiting **113**
  blood 116
Vulvovaginitis 141

Weight, figures 147
Wheezing 139
Whitlow, herpetic 124
Winter vomiting 115
Wound, infection of 13
Wounds *see* lacerations 45
Wringer injury **92**

X-ray examination
  abdomen 67, 77
  ankles 86
  arms 86
  cervical injury **86**, 134
  cervical spine 86
  data needed 9
  elbow 84, 86
  facial bones 74
  glass 50, 54
  hands 85
  head injury 70
  iron tablets 36
  limbs 84, 85
  mandible 74
  neck injury 86
  non-accidental injury 19, 20
  orbit 74
  requests 9
  rubber 53, 55
  scaphoid 86
  skull 71